100 PERFECT HAIR DAYS

Step-by-Steps for Pretty Waves, Braids, Curls, Buns, and More!

JENNY STREBE

CHRONICLE BOOKS

SAN FRANCISCO

First published in the United States of America in 2016 by Chronicle Books LLC.

Library of Congress Cataloging-in-Publication Data available.

ISBN: 978-1-4521-4335-4

Manufactured in China.

Cover designed by Anne Kenady

Publisher: Mark Searle
Editorial Director: Isheeta Mustafi
Commissioning Editor: Jacqueline Ford
Assistant Editor: Tamsin Richardson
Editor: Cath Senker
Design concept: Michelle Rowlandson
Book layout: Kate Haynes and Richard Peters
Illustrations: Jess Hibbert and Rob Brandt

10 9 8 7 6 5 4 3 2

Chronicle Books LLC
680 Second Street
San Francisco, CA 94107
www.chroniclebooks.com

IMAGE CREDITS

Front cover (clockwise from top): Hair Jenny Strebe, photography Tiffany Egbert, makeup Aeni Domme, model Dorthy Ha; Hair Anthony Lunam, photography Tiffany Egbert, makeup Stephanie Neiheisel, model Jess Hause; Hair Jenny Strebe, photography Tiffany Egbert, makeup Aeni Domme, model Bailey Harris.

Back cover (from top to bottom): Hair Jenny Strebe, photography Tiffany Egbert, makeup Stephanie Neiheisel, model Jess Hause; Hair Jenny Strebe, photography Tiffany Egbert, makeup Chelsea Cooper, model Chelsea Cooper; Hair Genevieve Reber, photography Tiffany Egbert, makeup Stephanie Neiheisel, model Amanda Shearer.

DEDICATION

This book is dedicated to my children, Magnolia and Indy.
May you always believe in yourselves and dream big. I love you.

CONTENTS

SECTION 1
HAIRSTYLES

CHAPTER 1
CASUAL

CHAPTER 2
OUT AND ABOUT

CHAPTER 3
SPORTY

CHAPTER 4
DRESS UP

CHAPTER 5
EXTRA SPECIAL

CHAPTER 6
PROBLEMS
& SOLUTIONS

INTRODUCTION

I have been a professional hairstylist for fifteen years, including six years as the educational director at a popular salon franchise. In that time, my work has been seen on TV and on the runway. I launched the blog Confessions of a Hairstylist because I loved seeing how good hair can inspire confidence in and empower women. Through my simple step-by-step tutorials, I have put an end to all bad hair days.

This book teaches you how to make the best of your hair. Over the years I have cut, styled, and colored every kind of hair, from fine, flat, and oily hair to wavy, curly, frizzy, and thick hair. Now I want to share my expertise and show you how to care for your own individual hair type and choose the right tools and products to make it look fantastic.

Section 1 offers one hundred different styles for you to create. I have tailored each look for specific hair types and textures. Discover new party looks, unique updos, brilliant braids, chic office styles, weekend top-knots, and many more. My goal is to help you make every day a perfect hair day.

Chapter 1 caters for casual days. It's full of great ideas for braids and stylish ways to wear your hair down when you want to keep it simple. Chapter 2 includes a range of buns, braids, and other ways to keep your hair tidy but stylish while you're on the go at work or running errands. Chapter 3 is for sporty days and events when you need your hair out of your face so you can be active but still want to look pulled together. Chapter 4 is designed for dress-up days when your hairstyle needs to impress as much as your outfit and includes modern versions of vintage styles and some fabulous updos. In Chapter 5 I go all out with styles for special days when you are heading to a formal function or want to make a statement—including unusual braids and upstyles with stunning shapes.

Each tutorial explains which hair type it's best for, how the style can help overcome hair problems, and how to prepare your hair to achieve the look. Illustrated step-by-step instructions show you how to create the style and photos demonstrate the finished result. You can do all the looks yourself but I've noted using a symbol with two faces where it may be helpful to have a partner. Want to try a specific look in the book but don't think you have the right hair type? The tutorials have insider information on how you can fake it! Turn fine hair into a thick braid, or tame flyaway and frizzy hair to produce a sleek, lustrous look.

Section 2, the Hair Spa, reveals the best hair care routines for every hair type, from washing, conditioning, and styling to problem solving and getting healthier hair. It's packed with information on selecting the top tools and products to make your hair look its very best.

So are you ready to get perfect hair? I've shared all my trade secrets in this book. Now you too can achieve salon-worthy hair in the comfort of your own home.

Let's get started!

Jenny Strebe

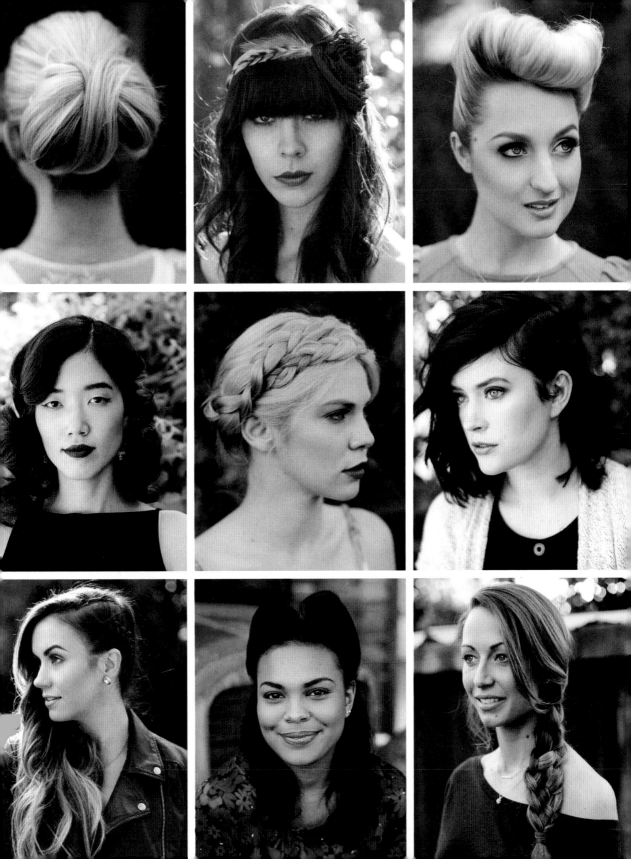

STYLE 101

Check out which number styles are perfect for your hair type.

 STRAIGHT
 FLAT
 THICK

CASUAL

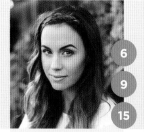 6 9 15

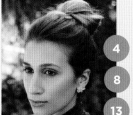 4 8 13

 6 10 14

OUT AND ABOUT

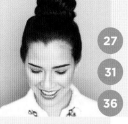 27 31 36

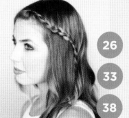 26 33 38

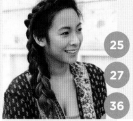 25 27 36

SPORTY

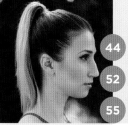 44 52 55

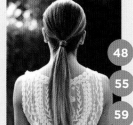 48 55 59

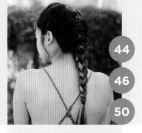 44 46 50

DRESS UP

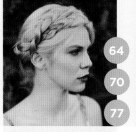 64 70 77

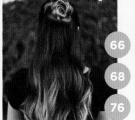 66 68 76

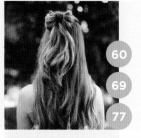 60 69 77

EXTRA SPECIAL

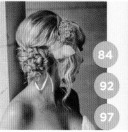 84 92 97

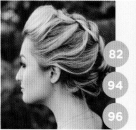 82 94 96

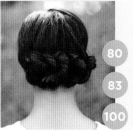 80 83 100

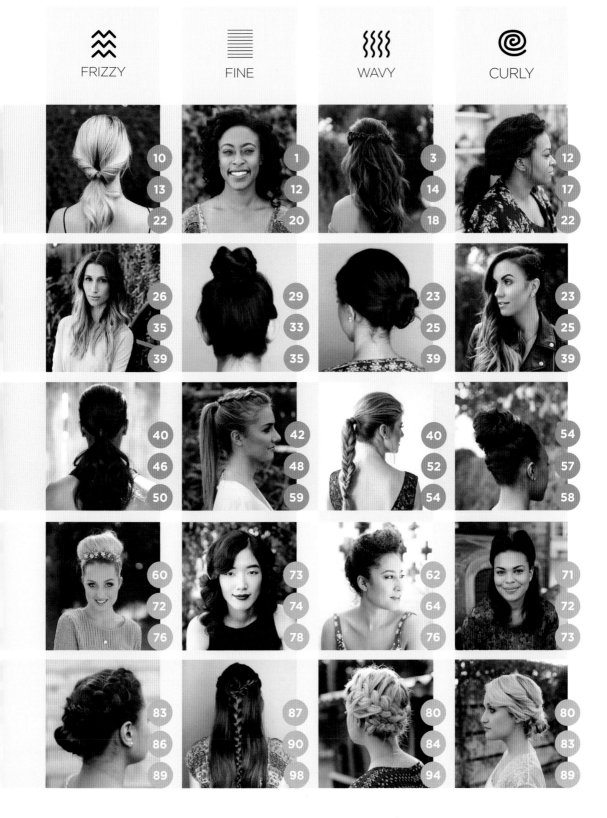

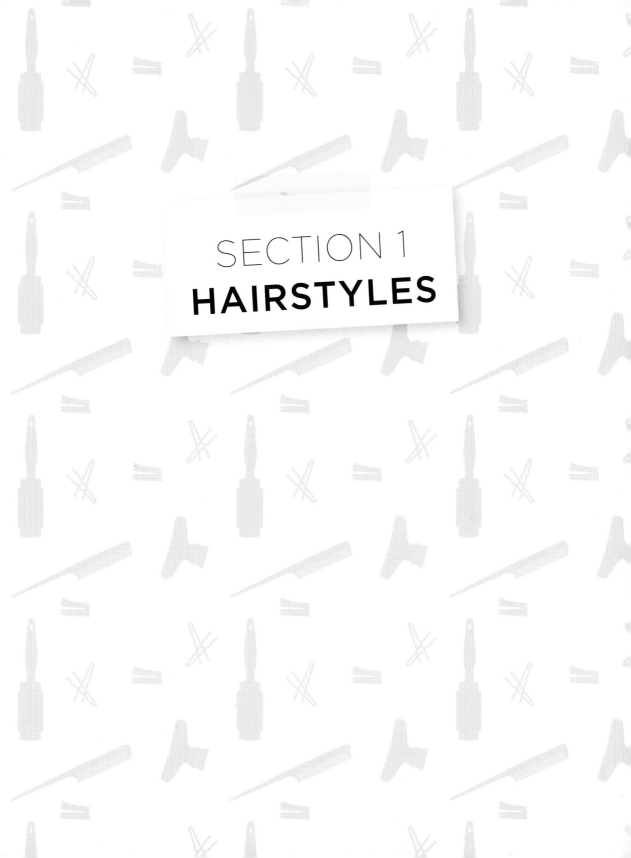

SECTION 1
HAIRSTYLES

CHAPTER 1
CASUAL

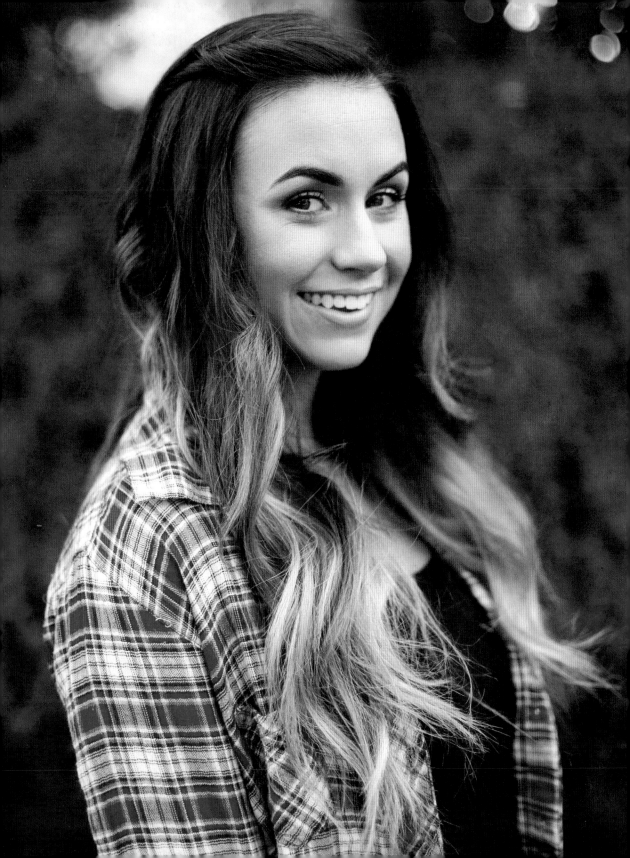

1. LOW LOOPED PONY

BEST FOR

 FINE

 STRAIGHT

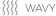 WAVY

This hairstyle is a variation on a low ponytail—the hair is looped into the hair elastic instead of being pulled all the way out. It is perfect for girls who have fine hair since when you pull back the hair, it actually makes the hair appear thicker. The low looped pony also works well with chemically textured, straight, and wavy hair because you'll be able to see the definition of the chic loop outside the ponytail. I recommend this hairstyle if you want to be low maintenance and crave healthier hair since you don't need to use any hot tools to create this look.

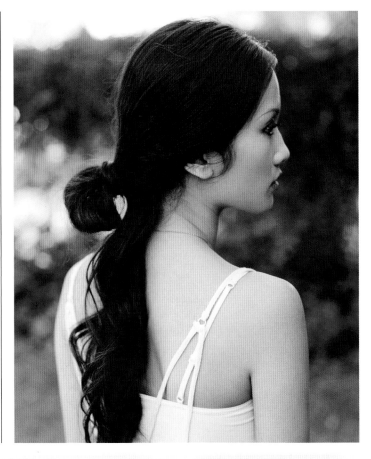

2. HALF-DOWN LOOPED PONY

Sometimes less is more, and in this case, the half-down looped pony is more! This variation is ideal for thick hair that is straight or wavy. The loop won't be too heavy because you have only half of your hair up yet it will look really dramatic. This style works best for hair that is on the straighter side because you will be able to see the loop clearly. If you have curly hair, throw some frizz control serum in your hair and use the straight hair tutorial (see page 42) to enjoy this look.

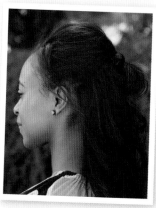

HOW TO DO IT

WHAT YOU NEED

- Hair elastic
- Bobby pin

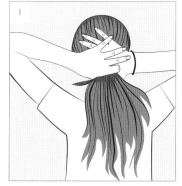

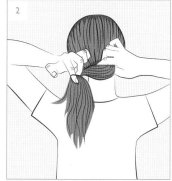

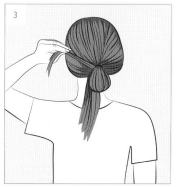

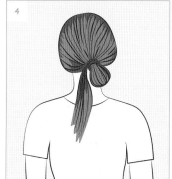

1. Gather all of your hair toward the nape of your neck.

2. Take a hair elastic and pull your hair through it as if you were making a normal ponytail.

3. Stop pulling your hair through when you have about 3 in (7.5 cm) of hair left out of the ponytail. This will create your "loop."

4. Take the elastic and go around your loop a few times, securing it tightly. To create a more polished look, take an inch (2.5 cm) of hair left out of the loop and take this section up and over the hair elastic. Secure the ends of this section with a bobby pin to hold it in place.

TIP

This hairstyle is ideal for one or two days after you've washed your hair. If your hair is recently washed, try grunging it up by adding a pomade or spray wax for some extra texture.

3. HALF-UP FISHTAIL BUN

BEST FOR

||||| STRAIGHT

§§§§ WAVY

≡≡≡ FINE

The half-up fishtail bun is similar to a top knot but instead you create a beautifully defined bun by wrapping a fishtail braid around your half-up ponytail. It is ideal for ladies who have straight to wavy hair. It also works best if your hair has minimal layers and is mid-length to long because you need sufficient length to be able to braid the top section. However, if you have short hair with some longer layers, you can make your fishtail bun from the long sections and leave out some hair at the front. This look is also great for girls with fine hair; by simply pulling out the braid, you will create more volume.

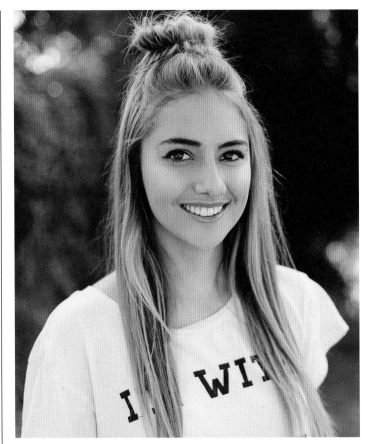

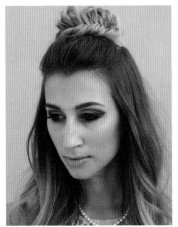

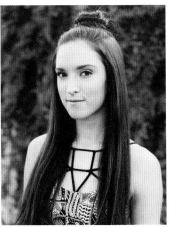

▶ **SEE ALSO**
Messy top knot,
page 18

HOW TO DO IT

WHAT YOU NEED

- Brush
- Hair elastics
- Bobby pins
- Medium-hold hairspray

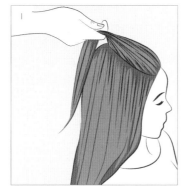

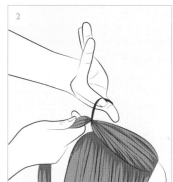

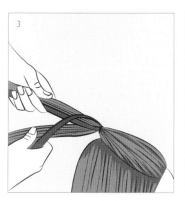

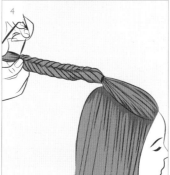

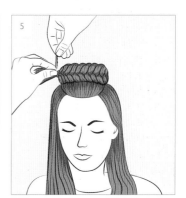

1. Brush all of your hair to ensure it is tangle free. Part the top of your hair off from the hairline to the top of your crown.

2. Secure the hair in a ponytail using a hair elastic at the crown of your head.

3. Create a fishtail braid using the ponytail (see page 38).

4. Continue to work the fishtail braid technique until you reach the ends of your hair and secure with a hair elastic.

5. Wrap the braided fishtail around the base of the ponytail and secure it with a couple of bobby pins. Finish off the look with medium-hold hairspray.

TIP

If your hair is fine, add volume by blow drying a mousse in your hair and adding some waves (see beach waves, page 24). This will create body so you can achieve a fuller fishtail bun.

4. MESSY TOP KNOT

BEST FOR

 CURLY

 FLAT

WAVY

Luckily, the messy top knot is still going strong—this simple style works well on second-day hair and is great for any girl on the go. It works well for mid-length to long hair because you need the length to wrap around the pony. It's good for hair that already has some texture to it, from wavy to curly—the texture will help add height and volume and keep it casual rather than sleek. If your hair is fine, try adding a thickening hair spray, throw in some thermal curls, and tease the roots so that you can fake thick hair.

 SEE ALSO
Half-up fishtail bun,
page 16

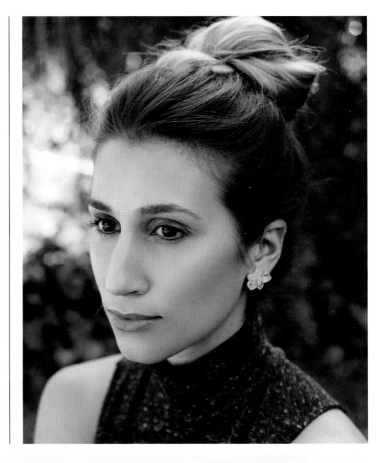

5. MESSY TOP KNOT WITH SCARF

Adding a scarf to your hair can give this hairstyle a completely different vibe, taking it from bohemian babe to vintage queen. To create this look, all you have to do is choose a large scarf, wrap it over your head around the hairline and tie it at the back.

To ensure your scarf stays in place, add a few bobby pins around the edges.

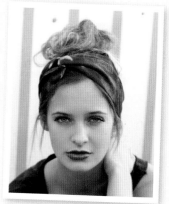

HOW TO DO IT

WHAT YOU NEED

- Hair elastic
- Comb
- Bobby pins
- Medium-hold hairspray

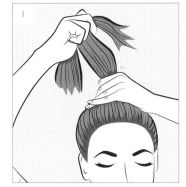
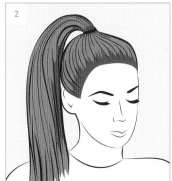
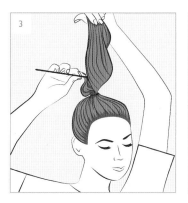
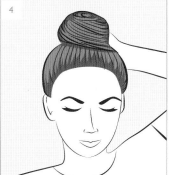
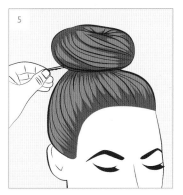

1. This style works best on unwashed hair—make sure it is completely dry. Create a very high ponytail by gathering all of your hair on top of your head.
2. Secure it with a hair elastic.
3. With a comb, slightly tease the ends of the hair down to the hair elastic.
4. Wrap the ponytail around the hair elastic.
5. Secure your hair with bobby pins. For extra hold, spray a medium-hold hairspray all over.

TIP

If your hair is really dirty or very fine textured, use dry shampoo all over before creating your top knot. This will help give your hair extra body and if it's dirty, it will give it a matte finish.

6. LOW ROPEBRAID

BEST FOR

 STRAIGHT

 THICK

The low ropebraid is simple and sweet and works for daytime and casual occasions. This hairstyle is good for the beginner braider and works best with mid-length to long hair that has few layers. It suits straight hair because you will be able to see the definition in the twists of the braid. It's great for days when you don't want to wash your hair; the natural oils will help smooth down any flyaways so you can achieve a tidy ropebraid. If your hair is frizzy, straighten it a little first by simply adding a bit of smoothing creme and blow drying it straight (see straight hair tutorial on page 42).

 SEE ALSO
Ropebraid bun, page 54

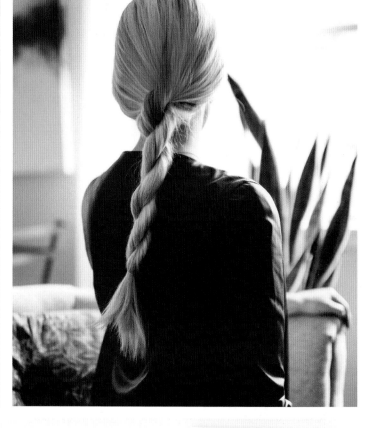

7. ROPEBRAID PONY

The ropebraid pony is also great for straight and second-day hair. Create a high ponytail by combing all the hair back toward the crown area and then securing with a hair elastic. Make a ropebraid inside your ponytail by splitting the hair in two sections. Twist the hair on the right side over to the right and take that section up and over to the left. Your left section is now on your right side, so twist it and take it over to the left side. Repeat this ropebraid technique until you get to the ends of the ponytail and secure with a hair elastic.

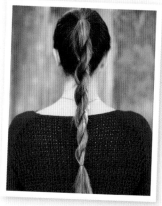

HOW TO DO IT

WHAT YOU NEED

- Brush
- Lightweight shine serum
- Hair elastic

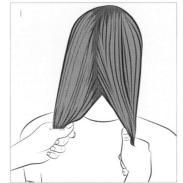
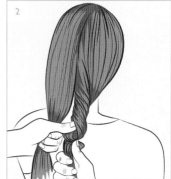
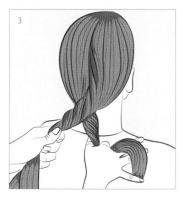
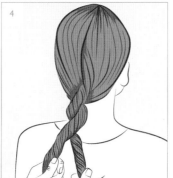
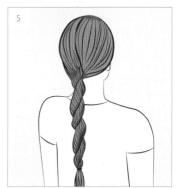

1. Brush your hair and apply a lightweight shine serum to help smooth any flyaways so that you will see the true definition of the ropebraid. Split the hair in half from your hairline down to the nape of your neck.

2. Twist the hair on your right side, going to the right.

3. Go up and over the left section with the twisted right section.

4. Take the section that is now on the right and twist it a few times to the right. Take this twisted section up and over to the left.

5. Continue with this pattern of twisting to the right and going up and over to the left until you don't have any more hair to work with. Secure the ends with a hair elastic.

TIP

When working with this technique, always twist to the right and go up and over to the left to keep the twists separate.

8. HALF-UP TOP KNOT

BEST FOR

≈≈≈ FRIZZY

≡≡≡ FLAT

The half-up top knot is simple to create and perfect for the casual yet trendy girl who has chemically textured hair. When your hair has been highlighted, it creates a chemical texture that will give it a lot of bulk, allowing the style to stay in place. It's a quick and simple way to add interest if you have flat hair too. And if you skip a hair wash the natural oils will help aid your dry ends, so the half-up top knot makes a good second-day style. If your hair isn't chemically textured, grit up your locks by blow drying some texture spray into your hair. This will create a full-looking top knot.

▶ SEE ALSO

Messy top knot, page 18

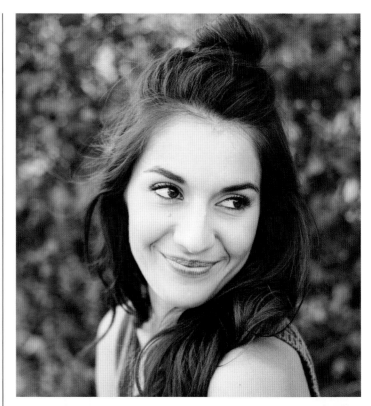

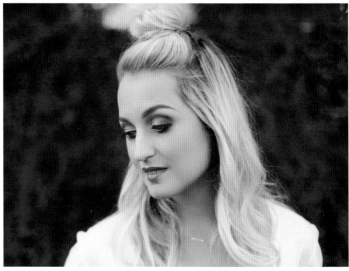

HOW TO DO IT

WHAT YOU NEED

- Comb
- Hair elastic
- Bobby pins
- Flexible-hold hairspray

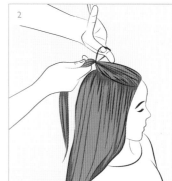

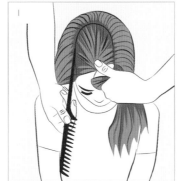

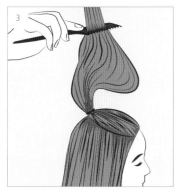

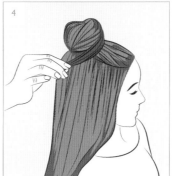

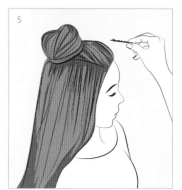

1. Create a large triangle section from each side of your hairline above your eyebrow, back to the crown.

2. Gather all the hair in your triangle section back to create a ponytail and secure into place with a hair elastic.

3. Since there is only a small amount of hair in your half-up top knot, I like to tease the hair aggressively to create bulk. Hold the hair straight up from the base of the ponytail, put the comb in halfway down, and tease the hair toward the base of the pony.

4. Wrap the teased hair around the base of your ponytail.

5. Secure the hair with bobby pins. Finish off the look with a flexible-hold hairspray.

TIP

Depending on how thick your hair is and how thick you want your top knot, feel free to take a larger or smaller triangle section at the beginning.

9. BEACH WAVES

BEST FOR

 FINE

 STRAIGHT

≀≀≀≀ WAVY

Calling all fine-haired females who suffer from flat and straight hair: this is the style for you! Sometimes straight hair can fall flat and hang from the roots, but you can easily transform lifeless hair by throwing some waves into it. This will instantly create fuller-looking hair, and fine hair will bounce up beautifully because it is not being weighed down. This style looks great if you have long hair that holds curls pretty well. If your hair is really thick and doesn't curl well, try adding a spray gel or a mousse before blow drying.

▶ **SEE ALSO**
Glamour waves, page 112

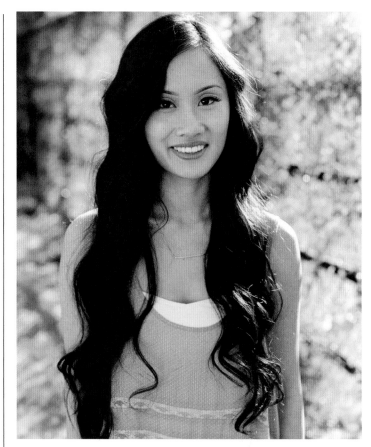

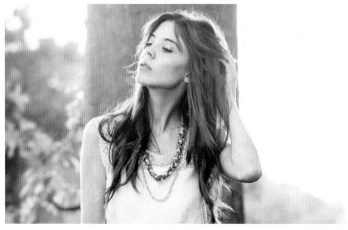

HOW TO DO IT

WHAT YOU NEED

- Clip
- Comb
- Curling iron (preferably 1 in [2.5 cm] or 1¼ in [3 cm])
- Flexible-hold hairspray

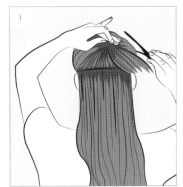

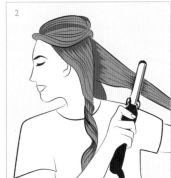

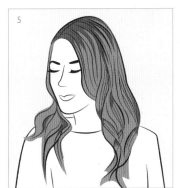

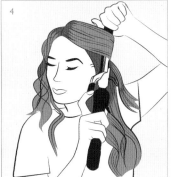

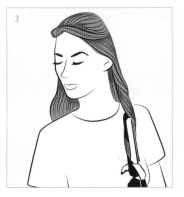

1. Start with 100 percent dry hair. Clip back your hair from ear to ear.

2. Start from the back of the head and work your way up. Take a small 1–2-in (2.5–5-cm) section (depending on the density of your hair). Using your curling iron, clamp down at the mid shaft of the hair.

3. Slowly ease the hair through the tong of the curling iron, then release the hair. By doing this, you are only curling the middle section of the hair, leaving the ends a bit looser.

4. Work this same technique at the top of the head.

5. Clip back sections and curl your hair until you have no more hair to work with. Use a flexible-hold hairspray to finish and lightly brush out your hair with your fingers to give a soft, tousled look.

TIP

If your hair is very thick or quite curl resistant, use flexible-hold hairspray before curling your hair. Spray it onto each section of hair from approximately 8-10 in (20-25 cm) away.

10. WAVES WITH A TWIST

BEST FOR

 THICK

 FRIZZY

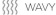 WAVY

To create this simple hairstyle, you take soft, beautiful curls and jazz them up by adding a simple twist. This look is great if you're on the go because the twist allows you to keep your hair out of your face while still looking styled. It's also a great option if you have have extremely thick hair with a wavy to frizzy texture. When you curl your hair with the iron, it will help tame any frizziness while adding lots of definition to your waves. If your hair is curl resistant, use a flexible-hold hairspray. If you have fine hair, apply some hair mousse and blow dry the opposite way to how your hair lies to achieve some fullness.

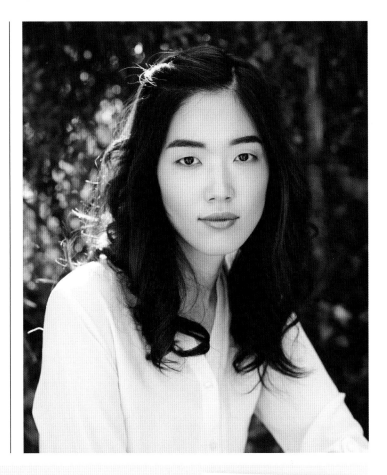

11. WAVES WITH FRENCH BACK BRAID

You can easily change the whole look of your waves with a twist by adding a soft French back braid. Take a small section of hair from your parting and divide it into three sections. Make a French braid (see page 80).

When you reach the top of your ear, continue with a simple three-braid technique until you get to the ends, and secure with a hair elastic.

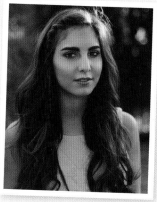

HOW TO DO IT

WHAT YOU NEED

- Comb
- 1¼-in (3-cm) curling iron
- Bobby pins
- Flexible-hold hairspray

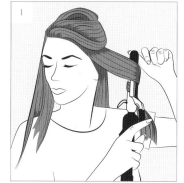

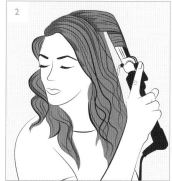

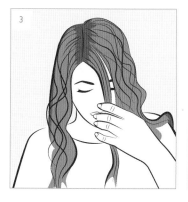

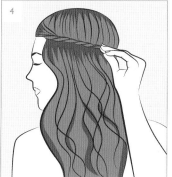

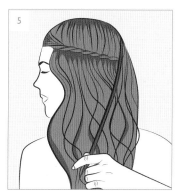

1. Start by sectioning off the hair from ear to ear around the back of your head, leaving a small section hanging down. Take 2–3-in (5–7.5-cm) sections of hair. Clamp down at the mid shaft of the hair and slowly ease the hair through the curling iron. When working with the sections around the face, curl away from the face.

2. Repeat this curling technique around the whole head. Lightly brush out with your fingers to add separation to the curls.

3. Part your hair on the side and separate out a triangle section about 3 in (7.5 cm) wide. If your hair is very thick, take a 2-in (5-cm) section.

4. Twist the hair going away from the face and wrap the section back. Take a bobby pin and pin it upward. If your hair is thick, try using two bobby pins and criss cross them.

5. Take the section of hair above the bobby pins and lay it over the top. Use hairspray to finish.

TIP

This style is great as a second-day hairstyle. Apply some dry shampoo at the roots before you start. The dry shampoo will give your roots a matte finish, making your hair appear like it is freshly washed.

12. NATURAL CURLY HAIR

BEST FOR

 CURLY

FINE

 WAVY

Curly hair can be frustrating sometimes, but it can also create some of the most beautiful hairstyles. Knowing how to wear your hair curly is just as important as being able to create a beautiful upstyle.

My natural curly hair style is ideal for girls who have fine- to medium-textured hair that is naturally wavy or curly with some natural bounce in it. When you already have some wave or curl you can really help enhance and define it by adding a few twists and utilizing some curl cream or amplifier. It's one of the easiest styles to create. Follow these simple steps so you can rock what your mama gave you in a matter of minutes.

▶ **SEE ALSO**
Waves with a twist, page 26

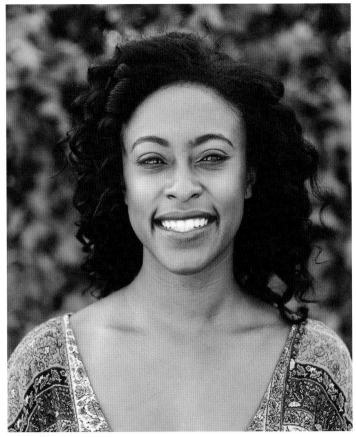

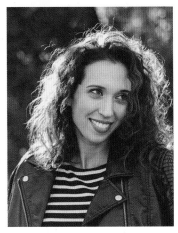

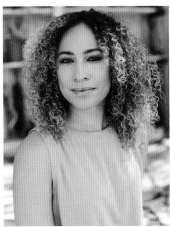

HOW TO DO IT

WHAT YOU NEED

- Curl cream or curl amplifier
- Wide-toothed comb
- Hair clip
- Blow dryer with diffuser attachment

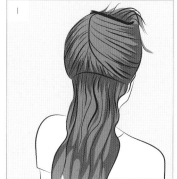

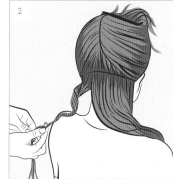

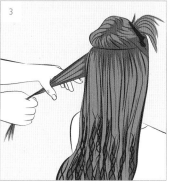

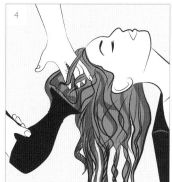

1. Apply a generous amount of curl cream or curl amplifier from roots to ends of towel-dried hair to saturate the hair. Starting at the nape of the neck, clip back a section of hair from ear to ear.

2. Below that section, take a 1–2-in (2.5–5-cm) section of hair and twist it to one side. Continue to take small sections and twist the hair gently. This allows the curls to clump together, creating a lot of curl definition. It also helps eliminate frizz.

3. Continue up to the top of the head, working the same technique. Take horizontal sections from one side of the hairline to the opposite side and twist small sections, until the hair is fully twisted.

4. Tip your head back and diffuse your hair in large sections using a blow dryer with a diffuser attachment on the low air setting. Put the ends of the curls in the diffuser and scrunch up the curls to the scalp.

TIP

The size of curls depends on the size of the twists. If you want tight curls, take smaller sections. Take larger sections to create bigger, fuller curls.

13. TOPSY-TAIL PONY

BEST FOR

 FINE

 FRIZZY

FLAT

A topsy-tail pony can make any ordinary ponytail look chic with little to no effort and it's perfect whether you're heading to go shopping or out with some friends. This style is great for second-day hair. It works best for fine-haired ladies who have chemically processed hair from color or highlights. When you pull the hair through your ponytail to create the topsy-tail, the slight roll it creates will make fine hair appear fuller, and the chemical texture will help it will stay in place. It's a successful style if you have flat hair because your twists at the back will help naturally create volume. If you lack a gritty texture from your hair being colored, try adding a bit of salt spray to your hair while damp and blow dry it in. This will coarsen up your hair. If you have short hair, try the half pony instead (see page 74), which is just as cute.

▶ **SEE ALSO**
Topsy-tail faux
braid, page 40

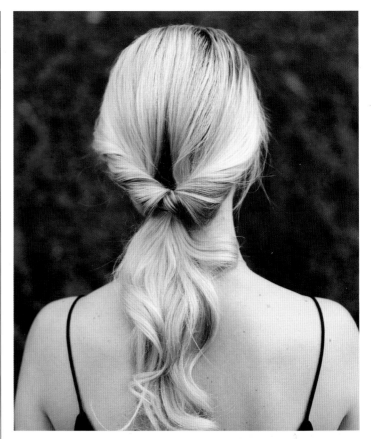

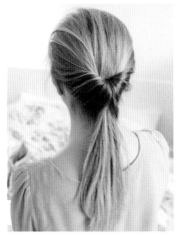

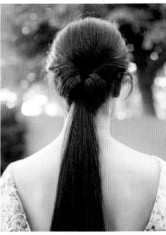

HOW TO DO IT

WHAT YOU NEED

- Comb
- Hair elastic

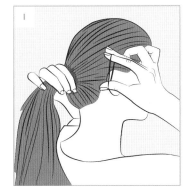

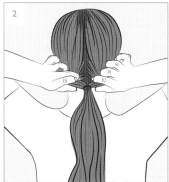

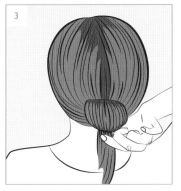

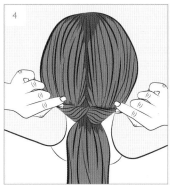

1. Comb your hair all the way through, toward the middle of the back of your head. Gather all of your hair at the back of your head and secure with a hair elastic.

2. Make a small gap between your hair elastic and your head by using your pointer finger and thumb to create a small opening behind the elastic band.

3. Take the ends of your ponytail, loop them through the small gap in your ponytail and pull through to the other side.

4. Once the hair is through the gap you will have an inside-out ponytail with attractive ridges on each side. You can pull at the sides of the twisted sections to add a bit more volume to the style.

TIP

You can also do a double topsy-tail by repeating the same technique an inch down from your original topsy-tail, or create a half topsy-tail by leaving some of your hair out of the first ponytail.

14. BROCADE BRAID HALF STYLE

BEST FOR

 STRAIGHT

 THICK

{{{{ WAVY

I'm all about easy hairstyles that make people wonder how you achieved such a stunning result, and the brocade braid (also known as the snake braid) is just that. This style is basically a three-strand braid, but when you hold on to two strands and gently pull up, the braid is completely transformed. I love this look because the result looks very difficult but it's actually pretty simple to achieve. The brocade braid hairstyle is ideal for women who have long, thick hair because when you create the brocade braid you need a lot of length to reach the back of your head. The hair needs to be thick so that you can see the true definition in the braid. If your hair isn't thick, you can still rock this do, but add a bit of thickening mousse in your locks before blow drying to help to bulk up your hair.

▶ **SEE ALSO**
Headband braid,
page 34

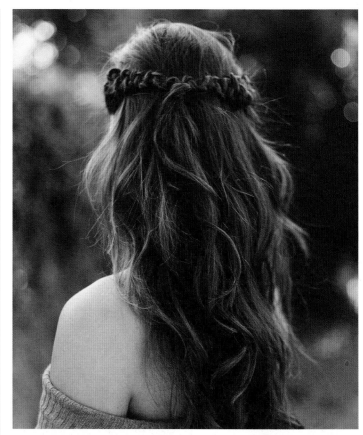

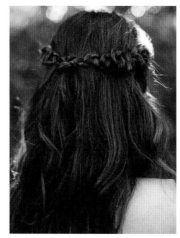

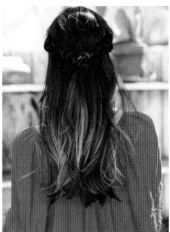

HOW TO DO IT

WHAT YOU NEED

- Brush
- Hair elastics
- Hair clips
- Shine spray (optional)

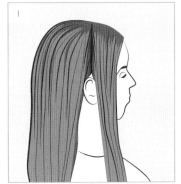

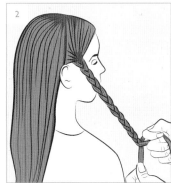

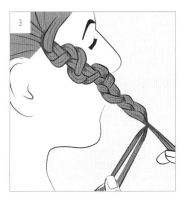

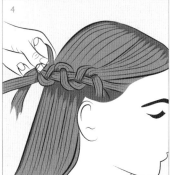

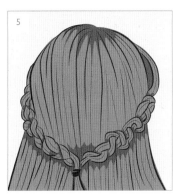

1. Start with dry hair. Section out the back of your hair from the top of your crown to right behind your ears to keep it out of the way.

2. Make a three-strand braid on the right (see page 51). When you have 2 in (5 cm) left, use your left hand to hold one of the strands of hair downward. Hold the other two with your right hand vertically.

3. Take the two strands you are holding with your right hand. Slowly pull them upward while you hold the third strand in your left hand. As you move the strands up, you will see the brocade pattern form.

4. Hold the ends of the hair tightly and continue braiding. Then brocade this section again as in Step 3 by pulling two of the strands upward.

5. When you reach the back of your head, secure the ends with a hair elastic and clip back. Do a brocade braid on the other side. Drape both braids across the back of your head, take out the hair elastics, and secure them together with one hair elastic.

TIP

If your hair is coarse or dry you may have difficulty with the braid traveling up. Try applying a shine spray beforehand to give your hair a silkier texture.

15. HEADBAND BRAID

BEST FOR

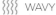 THICK

 STRAIGHT

WAVY

There's nothing cooler than being able to use your own hair to create a headband. To create a successful headband braid, you need the right hair type. This style works best if you have long hair and minimal layers because the braid goes right across the head. It's good for thick, straight or wavy hair because the braids are quite delicate and you want them to show up. If you have really fine hair and want to give this look a go, try plumping up your braid by gently pulling on each side to give it extra fullness.

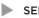 **SEE ALSO**
Brocade braid half style, page 32

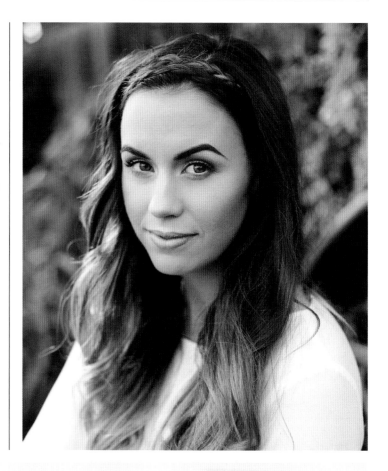

16. MULTI-BRAIDED HEADBAND BRAID

You will need long, thick hair to rock this do. Create a multi-braided headband braid by using the technique as above. With the remaining hair, create two ticker braids on each side. Wrap them across the front of your hairline, securing them in place with bobby pins. Feel free to get creative and use different types of braid technique, such as a ropebraid (see page 20) or a fishtail braid (see page 38).

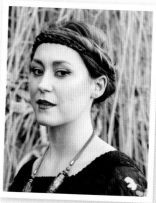

HOW TO DO IT

WHAT YOU NEED

- Hair clips
- Bobby pins
- Hair elastics
- Hairspray

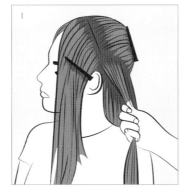

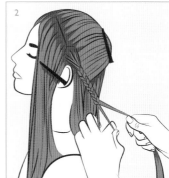

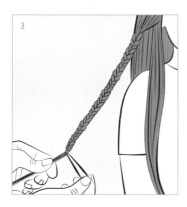

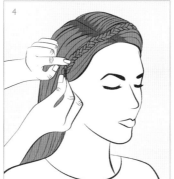

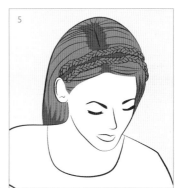

1. Start with dry hair. Clip back the front sections of hair in front of the ear and create a small 2–3-in (5–7.5-cm) rectangle section behind the ear. Clip the hair above it away for later.

2. Starting on the left, make a three-strand braid from behind the ear (see page 51) and secure with a hair elastic.

3. On the right side of your hair, create another three-strand braid and secure it with a hair elastic. Drop the clipped-back sections. Feel free to finish the loose hair how you see fit whether it be curly, light waves, or straight hair.

4. Take the braided sections over your head to the opposite side of your hair and bobby pin them in place.

5. Finish this look by hairspraying the braids into place.

TIP

You can get creative with this hairstyle and change up the whole look by simply changing the type of braid you do. Try fishtail braids for a very different finish.

17. TWISTED PONYTAIL

BEST FOR

 CURLY

THICK

A ponytail is classic, but sometimes, the standard pony might feel a bit boring. The ponytail with a twist brings in a little edge and a different feel, yet your hair is still casually pulled back into a classic ponytail. Incorporating hair from the sides takes a bit of practice but it's easy once you get the hang of it. I love creating this look on wavy to curly hair with medium to thick texture because it really allows your twists to stand out. It's also ideal for long hair so the hair left out of the ponytail hits your collarbone. You can still wear this style if your hair is extremely curly, but the twists won't be as well defined.

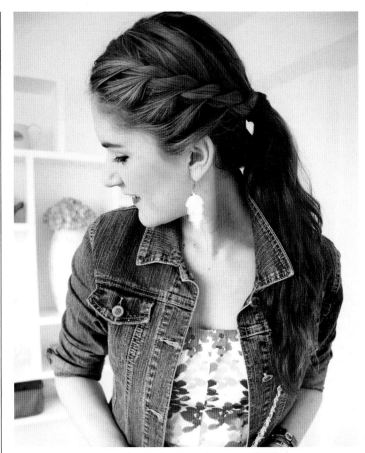

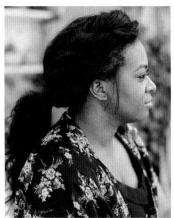

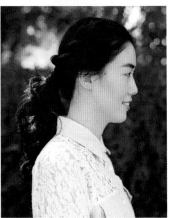

▶ **SEE ALSO**
Lace braid with waves, page 64

HOW TO DO IT

WHAT YOU NEED

- Comb
- Bobby pin
- Hair elastics
- Medium-hold hairspray

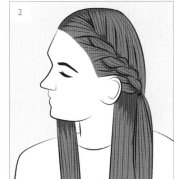

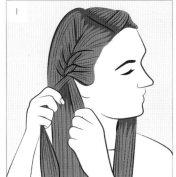

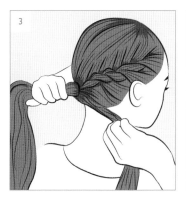

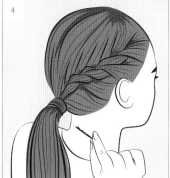

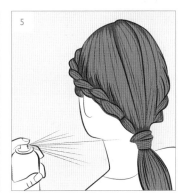

1. Separate the hair on the right side of your head into two sections and make a ropebraid along your hairline (see page 20). For this ropebraid technique, you connect the hair as you work down the side of the hairline. So every time you do a twist, incorporate some hair from above or below.

2. Continue until you get to right behind the ear and secure the ends with a hair elastic. Repeat this technique on the other side.

3. Gather all the hair left out of the ropebraids and create a low ponytail (see page 76). Secure it with a hair elastic. Use two if your hair is very thick.

4. Take a ¼-in (0.75-cm) section of hair from underneath the ponytail, wrap it around the hair elastic, and bobby pin the ends into the bottom of the ponytail.

5. For hold, use a medium-hold hairspray.

TIP

If your hair is really fine and your twists are small, you can gently pull on them before securing them into the ponytail. This will make your twists appear fuller.

18. FISHTAIL BRAID

BEST FOR

 FINE

 STRAIGHT

 WAVY

The fishtail braid is a classic. It's one of the easiest braids once you get the hang of it. This style can be worn in several different ways but the classic way is straight down your back. I love this look on girls with long, straight to wavy hair. It works beautifully for fine hair because you can pull on each side of the fishtail to give instant thickness. My thick-haired and curly-haired friends can easily achieve this look as well—blow dry your hair straight so it's smoother and skip the stage where you plump up the braid so it's not overly big.

 SEE ALSO
Fishtail pony, page 82

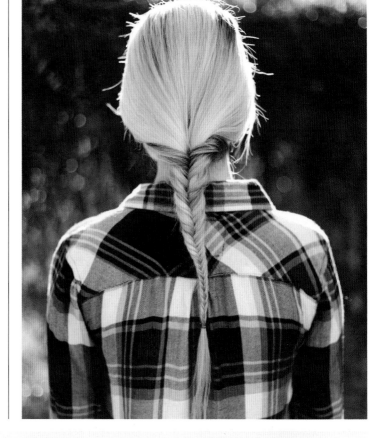

19. FISHTAIL BRAID UPDO

You can turn your fishtail braid into an elegant updo in minutes. This look is great for thick, straight hair—you will be able to see the definition of the braid and achieve a great upstyle look. Start by pulling on your braid gently to loosen it. Take the hair below the nape of the neck and tuck it under and into your braid and secure it in place with bobby pins. Finish off the look with medium-hold hairspray.

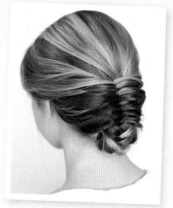

HOW TO DO IT

WHAT YOU NEED

- Comb or brush
- Shine serum
- Hair elastics
- Scissors

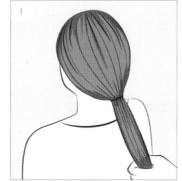

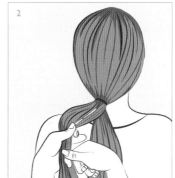

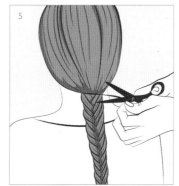

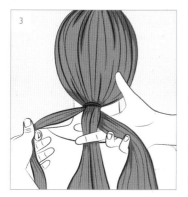

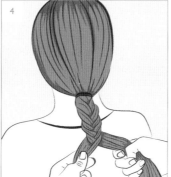

1. Use a shine serum from the middle of well-combed hair down to the ends. Comb all of your hair back to the nape of the neck, gather it, and loosely secure a hair elastic.

2. Divide your hair in half. Take a small section of hair from the right side and take it up and over into the left side.

3. Now take a small section of hair from the left side and go up and over to your right side.

4. Continue working this technique, working from right to left, until you get to the ends and you have about 1 in (2.5 cm) of hair left. Secure your hair with a hair elastic.

5. Carefully cut out the first hair elastic with scissors. To finish off the look, gently pull on each side of the braid to plump it up.

TIP

For a boho fishtail, plump out the braid but also hairspray it a little and massage it with the palms of your hands. This will create a really soft texture with little pieces hanging from the braid.

20. BOHO TOPSY-TAIL SIDE BRAID

BEST FOR

 FINE

 STRAIGHT

 WAVY

The boho topsy-tail side braid is the perfect style for fine hair since the topsy-tails give the appearance of thicker hair, and it works best if your hair is straight or wavy. It will suit you well if you have silky locks, which will make it easy to create the topsy-tails. This style is also ideal if you have very long hair so you can make a dramatic side braid.

▶ **SEE ALSO**
Topsy-tail pony,
page 30

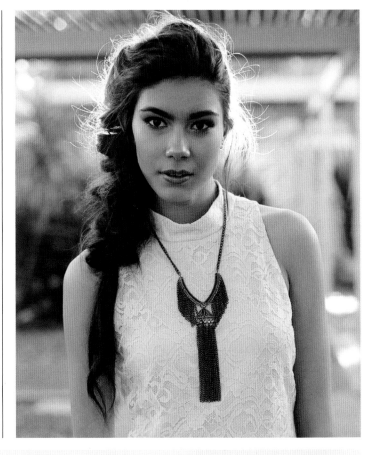

21. TOPSY-TAIL FAUX BRAID

This braid is perfect for novice braiders. It works beautifully for long, thick, silky hair. Create a ponytail and make topsy-tails as for the boho topsy-tail side braid. When you reach the nape of your neck, continue making topsy-tails until you get to a few inches away from the ends. Secure with a hair elastic. For added fullness in your style, gently pull on the sides of each topsy-tail.

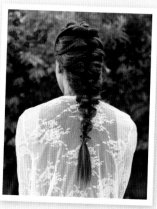

HOW TO DO IT

WHAT YOU NEED

- Brush
- Hair elastics
- Shine spray

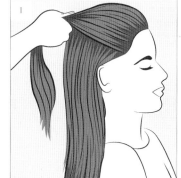

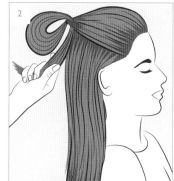

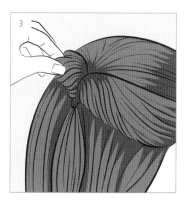

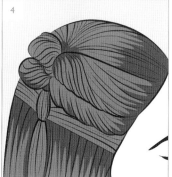

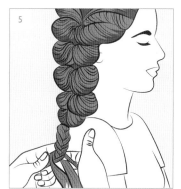

1. Brush your hair to the desired side. Make an off-center triangle parting from the high recession on the right of your head toward the opposite side near your ear.

2. Make a small ponytail about an inch (2.5 cm) away from your crown toward the right side and create a small topsy-tail (see page 30).

3. Aggressively pull on both sides of the topsy-tail to make it fuller.

4. Section the hair from each side of your hairline to about an inch under your first topsy-tail and make another one. Repeat this technique down the right side of the head until you reach the nape and secure the ends with a hair elastic.

5. Make a fishtail braid (see page 38) until 3 in (7.5 cm) of hair remains and secure with a hair elastic. Gently tug on the braid to make it fuller. Finish off with some shine spray to smooth any unwanted frizz.

TIP

If your hair is really thick you can still achieve this style, but instead of aggressively pulling the sides of the topsy-tails, gently tug so they are not too full.

22. STRAIGHT HAIR

BEST FOR

 FRIZZY

 CURLY

{{{{ WAVY

Knowing how to properly straighten your hair is a must. It's a classic that will never go out of style. This technique involves blow drying your hair and touching it up with a flat iron. It's easy to achieve with a little practice. The style is ideal for any girl who has some unwanted wave, frizz, or curl to her hair and wants to achieve a straighter and sleeker appearance. If you have naturally curly hair and want to wear a style such as the low chic pony (see page 86) or the low rolled updo (see page 148), you can straighten your hair first to provide a good foundation. If your hair is already straight and you're looking for some extra straightness, all you have to do is add a heat protectant from mid-shaft down and skim through your hair with a flat iron, and you're good to go.

▶ **SEE ALSO**
Hair products,
page 166

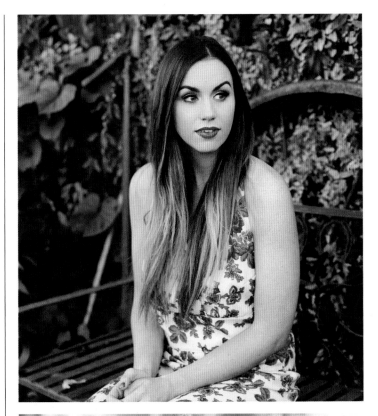

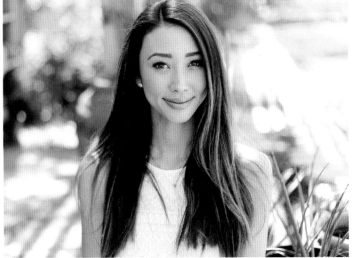

HOW TO DO IT

WHAT YOU NEED

- Hair straightening serum
- Comb
- Hair clip
- Round brush
- Blow dryer with nozzle
- Flat iron
- Shine serum

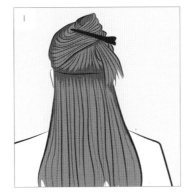

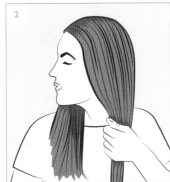

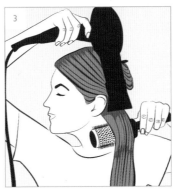

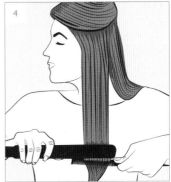

1. Apply a generous amount of hair straightening serum to combed, towel-dried hair. Divide your hair from ear to ear; clip back the top.

2. Take the round brush underneath a section of hair. Make sure the section is smaller than your round brush, and if your hair is extremely curly or frizzy, then take a smaller section.

3. With the blow-dryer nozzle pointing down, slowly blow dry your hair from the roots to the ends. Use plenty of tension to pull your hair straight and down. You may have to do this a few times until the hair is 100 percent dry. Dry all the sections of hair.

4. For extra chicness, touch up each section from the roots to the ends with the flat iron. Comb each section first, then skim the flat iron through the hair. Once your hair is dry, use some shine serum to smooth the hair.

TIP

It's important to always work with a nozzle on the blow dryer. Make sure to point it down and almost parallel with your hair section. This will help eliminate frizz and smooth any flyaways.

CHAPTER 2
OUT AND ABOUT

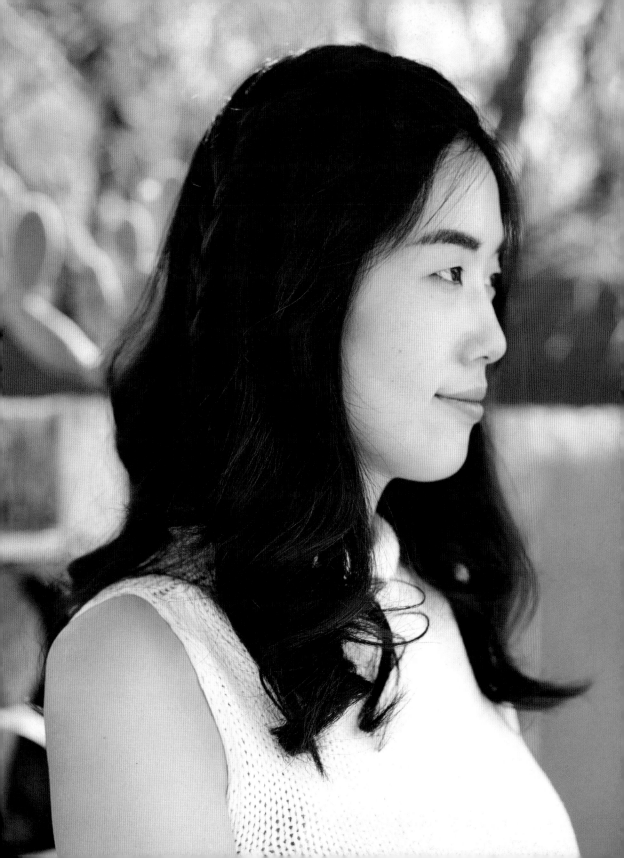

23. TWISTED CHIGNON

BEST FOR

〰〰 WAVY

◎ CURLY

The twisted chignon is one of the simplest hairstyles and it's a classic that will never go out of style. It looks best on collarbone to mid-length hair because you only need enough hair to wrap into a bun once or twice. I love this look on girls who have a bit of wave or curl to their hair so that when you twist the hair into a bun, the hair bends into the chignon. Sometimes, women with straighter hair have problems with this style because it can stick straight out. I recommend adding a bit of curl to the hair before you start.

 SEE ALSO
Low braided bun, page 52

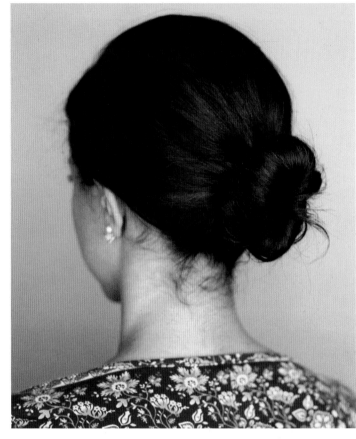

24. TRIPLE TWISTED CHIGNON FAUX HAWK

The triple twisted chignon is edgy and chic and suits the same hair types as the twisted chignon. It is achieved by doing three twisted chignons down the center of the head. First, divide your hair into three equal sections from the sides of your hairline across to the other side. Clip back two sections. Working with one section at a time, create a ponytail and twist the hair until it ravels to create a twisted bun. Secure the hair around your ponytail in place with bobby pins. Use hairspray to finish.

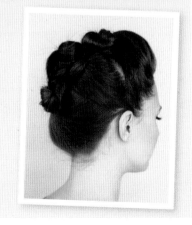

HOW TO DO IT

WHAT YOU NEED

- Brush
- Hair elastic
- Bobby pins
- Shine serum
- Firm-hold hairspray

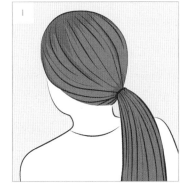

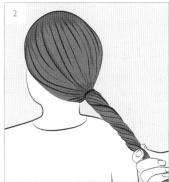

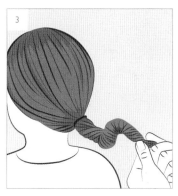

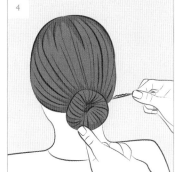

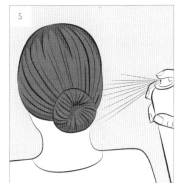

1. Start with completely dry hair. Apply a little shine serum to give your twisted chignon a polished look. Brush all the hair back to an inch (2.5 cm) above the nape of your neck. Gather it tightly and secure the hair with a hair elastic (use two if your hair is thick).

2. Take the hair that is out of the tail and twist it to the end.

3. Twist it further until the twists bunch up and start to create the bun shape.

4. Wind your twisted hair around the hair elastic and pin it in place using bobby pins.

5. To finish off the look, use a firm-hold hairspray.

TIP

To eliminate any lumps and bumps, stick the end of a weaving comb in your hair around the hairline and smooth toward the back of your ponytail.

25. PONY KNOT

BEST FOR

 CURLY

 THICK

 WAVY

The pony knot is the perfect alternative to a ponytail. It's simple to achieve but will definitely impress your friends. The pony knot works best on long hair so that after you create your knot, you have plenty of hair left out for the ponytail. It looks best on hair that is slightly wavy to curly. This is because when your hair has some wave to it, your pony knot is less likely to slip out. If your hair isn't wavy or curly, you can throw some curls in your hair before starting (see natural curly hair on page 28), and use some dry shampoo to add texture. Then you will easily be able to achieve this style.

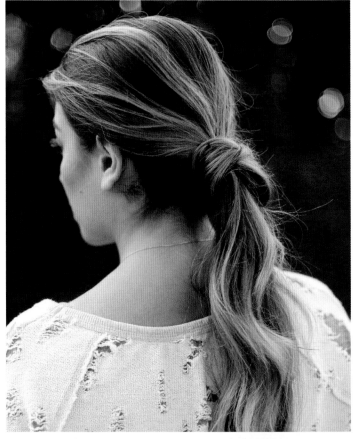

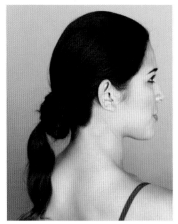

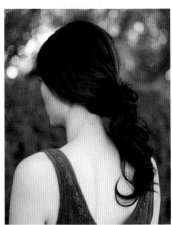

SEE ALSO
Low pony, page 76

HOW TO DO IT

WHAT YOU NEED

- Brush
- Hair elastic
- Bobby pins
- Medium-hold hairspray

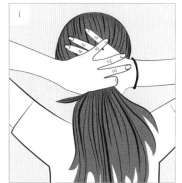

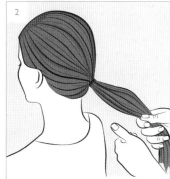

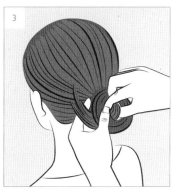

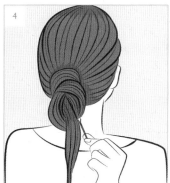

1. Start with completely dry, well-brushed hair. Gather your hair loosely toward the nape of your neck and comb through with your fingers to give it an undone soft texture.

2. Create a low, loose ponytail and secure with a hair elastic.

3. Make a simple knot by creating a large loop near the base of the ponytail and pulling the ends of the ponytail through the loop. This will create a large knot at the base of your ponytail.

4. Use a bobby pin or two (or more if you have very thick hair) underneath the base of the knot to secure it into place. Finish off the look with a medium-hold hairspray.

TIP

If your hair is extremely thick, the knot might not hold. You can just use the top half of your hair to make the ponytail so the knot will be smaller.

26. MESSY SIDE BRAID

BEST FOR

 FLAT

 FINE

 FRIZZY

Nothing says simple and sweet like a messy side braid. This style is very versatile and makes a great casual look for the working day or a relaxing weekend. You can dress up the messy side braid by adding a simple jewel embellishment or by adding a floral piece for something more bohemian. This style is perfect for second-day hair. When your hair is a little dirty, it will look disheveled yet still defined because your natural oils will help smooth any flyaways. You can wear this look if you have frizzy hair; your natural frizziness will add to the loose, casual appearance of the braid. I also prefer this style on hair that is fine to medium textured; your hair won't be weighed down, and you will get plenty of volume.

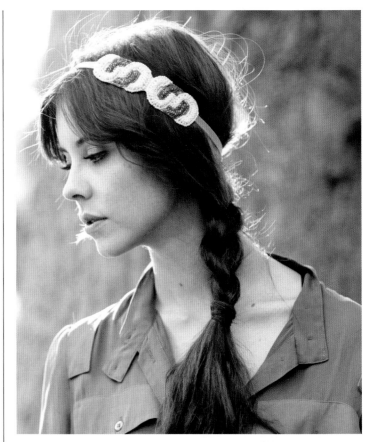

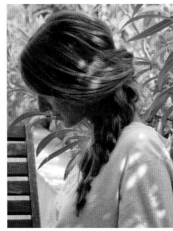

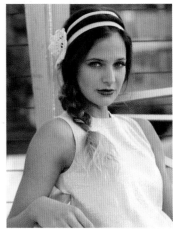

▶ **SEE ALSO**
Boho topsy-tail side braid, page 40

HOW TO DO IT

WHAT YOU NEED

- Comb
- Hair elastic
- Hairspray (optional)

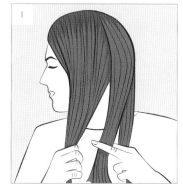

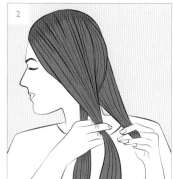

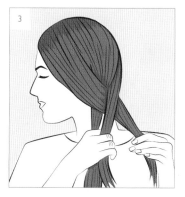

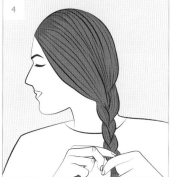

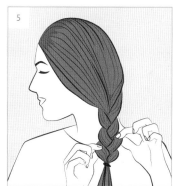

1. Start with dry hair, either clean or dirty. Sweep all your hair to the desired side and divide it into three sections.

2. Take the section on the left and cross it up and over to place it in the middle.

3. Take your section to the right and cross it up and over to place it in the middle.

4. Repeat this technique, switching from left to right, until you get to the ends.

5. Secure the ends with a hair elastic. To create a messy texture, gently pull on each strand to plump up your braid.

TIP

If you want your hair to be very messy, massage some of your hair out of the braid to create some wispy pieces. Use hairspray if needed to keep the wisps in place.

27. TOP BRAIDED BUN

BEST FOR

 THICK

 STRAIGHT

Impress all of your friends with the easiest updo ever! All you need to be able to do is a simple three-strand braid. This style can look casual or elegant—you could wear it for a barbecue or to attend a fancy dinner. I love this look on thick hair. Sometimes thick hair in updos can be weighed down and heavy, but if you braid your thick tresses first, it will help hold your hair into place without the hassle of a lots of bobby pins. It's best for mid-length hair so that you have enough hair to wrap around your pony once or twice.

▶ **SEE ALSO**
Ropebraid bun,
page 54

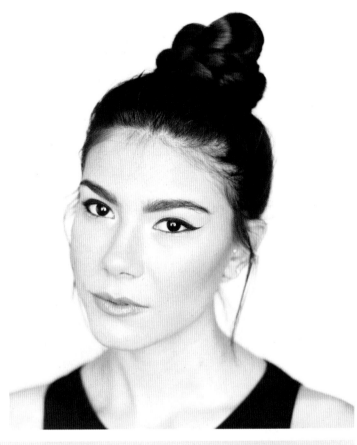

28. LOW BRAIDED BUN

The low braided bun is another very straightforward updo yet it can pack a lot of punch. To create this hairstyle, brush all of your hair to the back of the neck and secure the hair with a hair elastic. Then create a simple three-strand braid (see page 51) inside your ponytail and secure the ends with a hair elastic. Wrap your braid around the base of your ponytail to create a bun shape and pin into place with bobby pins. Finish off the look with medium-hold hairspray.

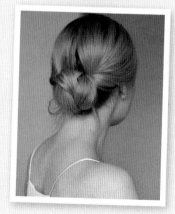

HOW TO DO IT

WHAT YOU NEED

- Hair elastics
- Bobby pins
- Firm-hold hairspray

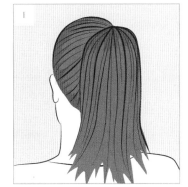

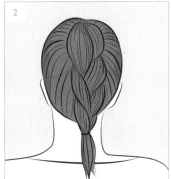

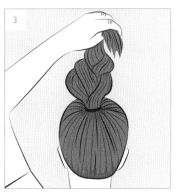

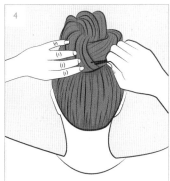

1. Loosely pull all your hair to the crown of the head and secure with a hair elastic to create a high ponytail. If your hair is really thick, add another elastic for extra hold.

2. Divide the hair into three sections and make a simple three-strand braid (see page 51). Secure the ends with a hair elastic.

3. If your hair is fine textured and you want your bun to appear thicker, simply tug at the strands to plump up your braid.

4. Wrap the braid around your high ponytail and bobby pin it into place. If you are going to wear this hairstyle for a night on the town, finish it off with some firm-hold hairspray.

TIP

If you want a voluminous bun, aggressively backcomb at the roots then comb the top layer out and secure it into your pony before doing your braid.

29. ROPEBRAID BUN

BEST FOR

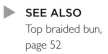 WAVY

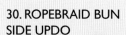 FINE

The ropebraid bun is a great hairstyle for the girl on the go who still wants to look fashionable. I love this hairstyle because it's simple, chic, and only takes minutes. This look is best on hair that is long with a fine texture to allow you to have a long, slender ropebraid. This do is also ideal for ladies who have a wave to their hair. The hair will naturally twist into the ropebraid so you won't have a lot of straight pieces sticking out. But don't worry, straight-haired friends; simply add a bit of wave to your hair before getting started.

▶ **SEE ALSO**
Top braided bun,
page 52

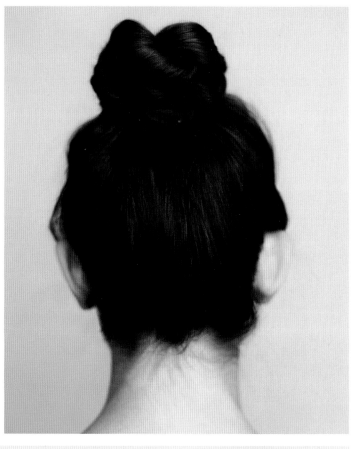

30. ROPEBRAID BUN SIDE UPDO

If a top-knot bun isn't your thing, you can easily use the ropebraid technique and turn your hair into a gorgeous ropebraid bun side updo. This look can be casual or elegant, depending on what you wear with it. I like this look on thick hair that is mid-length to long so you can create a really full side updo. Gather all of your hair into a side ponytail, and use the ropebraid technique as above, going toward your desired side. Wrap the ropebraid around the side pony and bobby pin it into place.

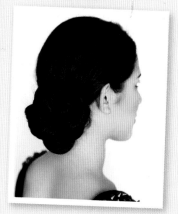

HOW TO DO IT

WHAT YOU NEED

- Brush
- Hair elastic
- Bobby pins
- Medium-hold hairspray

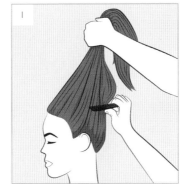

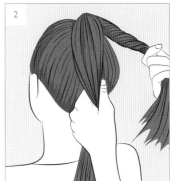

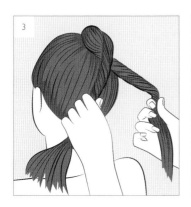

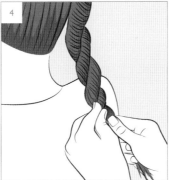

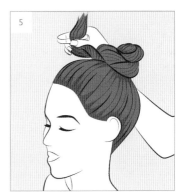

1. Brush your hair toward the crown of the head, gather all the hair together, and secure with a hair elastic to create a ponytail. If your hair is really thick, I suggest adding a second elastic.

2. Divide the hair left out of the ponytail in half. Twist the hair on the right side over to the right and up and over to the left. The section that was on your left side is your new right section.

3. Repeat the previous step by twisting the hair to the right, and take that section of hair up and over to your right. When you work this ropebraid pattern, it will allow the twists to stay separated, giving the ropebraid appearance.

4. Continue until you get to the ends and secure with a hair elastic.

5. Wrap the ropebraid around the base of the ponytail, securing it with bobby pins to create a bun. Finish off with a medium-hold hairspray.

TIP

If your hair is fine, and/or you want to create a larger ropebraid look, try spraying some dry shampoo in your hair beforehand. It will help create bulk and texture, making your hair appear fuller.

31. HIGH FISHTAIL BUN

BEST FOR

 STRAIGHT

 THICK

The fishtail bun is a fun yet sophisticated bun that is a spin-off from the fishtail ponytail. Once you've mastered the fishtail technique, it's easy to do. I'm obsessed with this style on girls who have thick, long hair which makes it possible to create a really large gorgeous bun. I also love this style on silky hair, which gives an elegant look. If your hair isn't naturally silky, try adding some shine serum to your locks before getting started as this will help smooth your flyaways and create a polished look.

▶ **SEE ALSO**
Top braided bun,
page 52

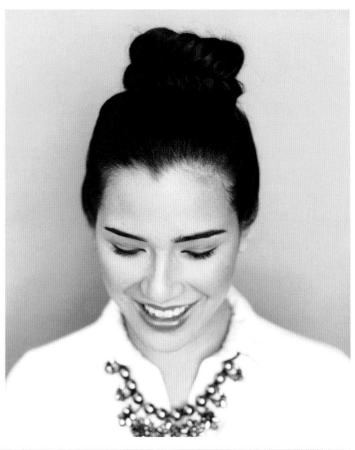

32. MULTI FISHTAIL BUN

If you really want to impress your friends, show up to happy hour with a multi fishtail bun. This style is a bit more avant-garde than your typical fishtail bun. I love this look with fine hair—you can pull the braids out for volume to make your hair appear thicker. The style is also good for chemically textured hair because it gives the style hold. To create this style, simply pull your hair up into a high ponytail, create four or five small fishtail braids within your ponytail, and wrap each individual fishtail braid around your hair elastic, securing with bobby pins as you go.

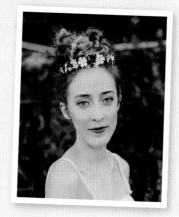

HOW TO DO IT

WHAT YOU NEED

- Brush
- Hair elastics
- Medium-hold hairspray

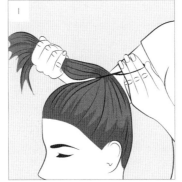

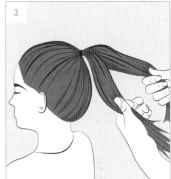

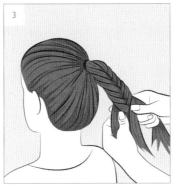

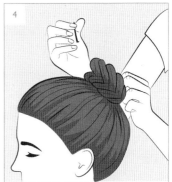

1. Brush all of your hair toward the high crown of your head, gather the hair, and create a ponytail, securing it with a hair elastic. If your hair is really thick, I suggest that you use two hair elastics.

2. Divide the hair inside your ponytail into two.

3. Follow the fishtail braid technique (see page 38) and secure the ends with a hair elastic.

4. Take your fishtail braid and wrap it around the top hair elastic, securing it in place with bobby pins as you go. Finish off this look by spraying a medium-hold hairspray all over.

TIP

To tame flyaways from layers or breakage, you can liberally spritz shine spray all over your braid and bun. This will create a sleek look.

33. SOCK BUN

BEST FOR

 FINE

 FLAT

The sock bun hairstyle is perfect
for ladies who have fine textured
hair—the sock-bun donut acts as
hair padding to make the hair
appear fuller. Anyone can wear
a sock bun, but the thicker and
longer the hair, the bigger the
bun. This style works best for
hair that is at least collarbone
length as you need enough
length to pull up and fit around
the bun. It is also great as a
second-day hairstyle because
having a little bit of extra grit
to your hair will help hold it
into place. It's an easy do
for beginners.

▶ **SEE ALSO**
  Bouffant bun,
  page 94

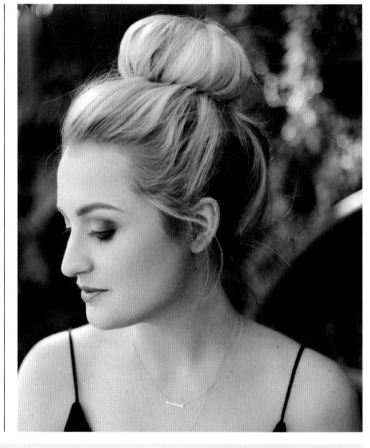

34. LOW SOCK BUN UPDO

A low sock bun updo is
a great alternative to the
regular sock bun for fine hair
since the sock bun adds lots
of volume to your bun. To
create the bun, secure your
ponytail at the nape of your
neck instead of the top. Then
simply wrap the ends of the
ponytail in the sock bun and
roll it toward the nape of
your neck. Once the sock
bun has reached the low
pony, secure it into place
with bobby pins. Finish off
this look with a medium-
hold hairspray.

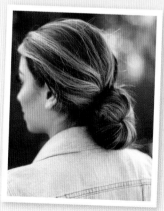

HOW TO DO IT

WHAT YOU NEED

- Comb
- Hair elastic
- Sock-bun donut
- Bobby pins
- Firm-hold hairspray

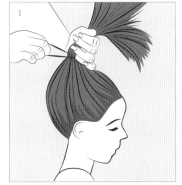

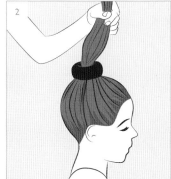

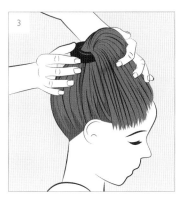

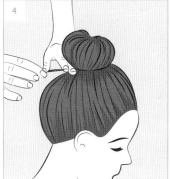

1. Comb all of the hair up toward the high crown area and secure with a hair elastic to create a very high ponytail.

2. Place the sock-bun donut around the ponytail at the base of your pony, leaving the loose hair out.

3. Take the loose hair from the pony and wrap it evenly over the sock-bun donut. Tuck the hair under the sock-bun donut.

4. Secure the tucked-in hair in place with bobby pins, pushing them into the sock bun near the scalp. Finish off the look with a firm-hold hairspray.

TIP

If you don't have a sock-bun donut, it's easy to make one! All you need to do is cut the end off a clean sock and roll into a round donut shape.

35. FLAT-IRON WAVES

BEST FOR

 FINE

 FRIZZY

Flat-iron waves give just the right amount of curl if you're trying to go for a messy rather than defined type of curl. You can easily throw a floral crown on this look to make it bohemian. These types of waves usually leave the hair with just a little bit of bend, with straighter ends. I love this style on hair that is on the longer side and fine to medium texture, but most importantly, hair that is prone to being frizzy. With this technique, you gently slide your hair through the flat-iron plate, which will instantly smooth any flyaways and frizz, leaving the hair smooth and soft. It takes a little time to get this technique right but it's well worth the effort.

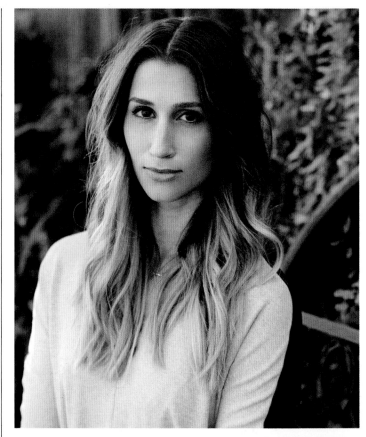

▶ **SEE ALSO**
Beach waves, page 24

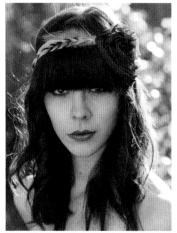

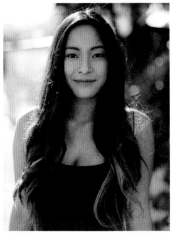

HOW TO DO IT

WHAT YOU NEED

- Hair clips
- Comb
- Flat iron
- Light hairspray if your hair doesn't hold very well

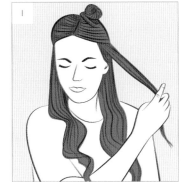

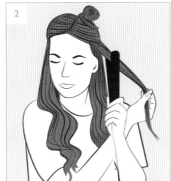

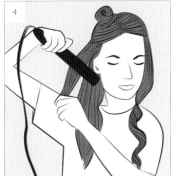

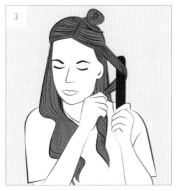

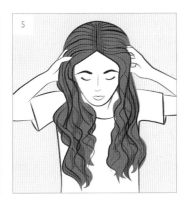

1. Start with 100 percent dry hair. Beginning at the nape of the neck, section out your hair in 1–2-in (2.5–5-cm) sections. Hairspray each section if your hair is curl resistant.

2. Clamp the flat iron down in the middle of a section.

3. Flip your wrist around so that the hair is wrapped around the iron.

4. Pull the flat iron straight out in a fast, steady movement and release when it gets to the ends. Repeat this technique, working from the nape of your neck up to the top of your head.

5. Run your fingers through your hair to comb out the curls and finish with hairspray if necessary.

TIP

If you want a rocker look, use spray wax in your hair while blow drying your hair on high heat. The heat will soften the wax and it will create lots of separation in the hair once you create the waves.

36. MERMAID SIDE DUTCH BRAID

BEST FOR

 THICK

 STRAIGHT

~~~~ WAVY

No one said that being a mermaid was easy, but once you've mastered this hairstyle tutorial, you'll have mermaid locks to be proud of. The side Dutch braid is an inverted side French braid, where you work the sections under-handed instead of over-handed. To create a plump, dramatic side Dutch braid, long, thick hair is ideal. The style looks best with straight to wavy hair so that you can see the definition of the braid. If your hair isn't very thick, use a salt spray and root lifter before you blow dry to make it appear a lot fuller.

▶ **SEE ALSO**
Dutch braid, page 90

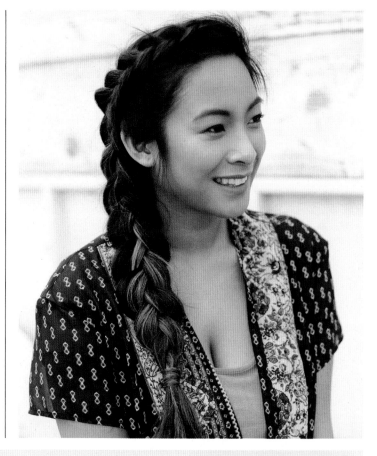

37. HALF DUTCH BRAID

The half Dutch braid is very similar to the mermaid side Dutch braid, but you don't have to incorporate all of your hair. I love this look with hair that is thick and has some wave to it. To create this style, simply clip the hair underneath that you don't want to incorporate into the braid and then release it once you have done your Dutch braid.

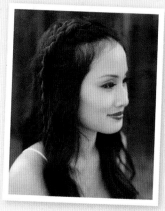

HOW TO DO IT

WHAT YOU NEED

- Comb
- Hair elastic

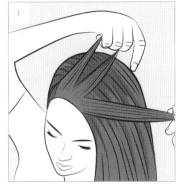
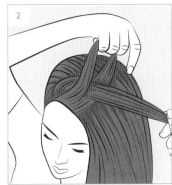
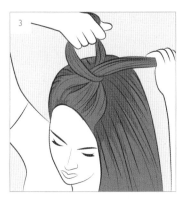
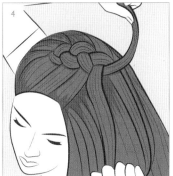
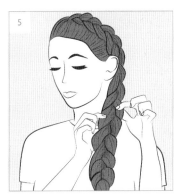

1. Take a 1–2-in (2.5–5-cm) section of hair at the hairline on one side and split it into three.

2. Begin your Dutch braid by bringing the right section under the middle, and the left section under the right. Then add some hair to the middle piece (now on the right side) and bring it under.

3. Repeat, adding in hair from the left side and bringing that section under into the middle.

4. You still add in hair from both sides with this braid, but you keep the braid close to your hairline along the side of your face. When adding in hair on the right, take sections from across the back of your head.

5. Once you've added all your hair to the braid, work a regular three-strand braid (see page 51). Secure the end with a hair elastic. Pull gently on each section of the braid to make it appear fuller.

TIP

If you have really fine textured hair, add some dry shampoo to your hair to add extra bulk to your locks.

38. LACE BRAID WITH WAVES

BEST FOR

 FLAT

 FINE

The lace braid with waves is a gorgeous alternative to a simple Dutch or French braid. To make a lace braid, you only incorporate hair into one side of the braid, which creates a beautiful yet delicate braiding design. This is a great hairstyle if you're growing out your bangs because it allows you to wear your hair out of your face while still looking stylish. It's perfect for girls who tend to have hair that falls flat, because it will add some interest. It works well for fine hair as well; the lace braid won't take any weight out of the hair or make the ends look sparse because it is placed on top of the hair. This is also a great look for mid-length hair—you don't need to have a lot of length since the braid travels across the top.

▶ **SEE ALSO**
Twisted waterfall braid, page 136

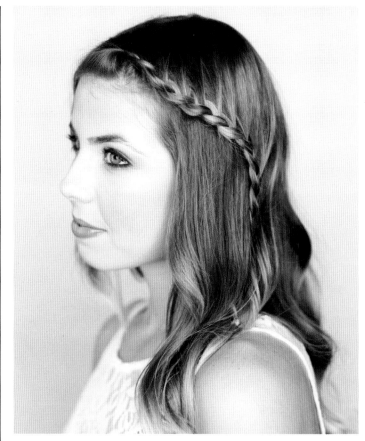

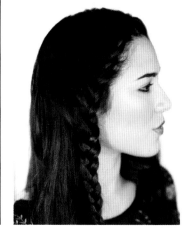

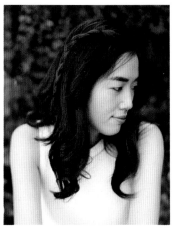

HOW TO DO IT

WHAT YOU NEED

- Brush
- Shine serum
- Hair elastic
- Medium-sized curling iron

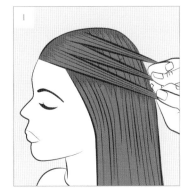

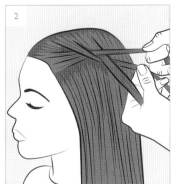

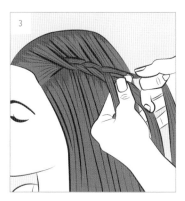

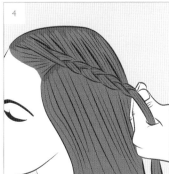

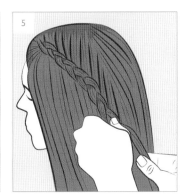

1. Brush out your hair with a little shine serum to make it smooth. Starting on the desired side, take a small section of hair at your parting and hairline and create three small sections of hair.

2. Cross the section from the hairline under the middle section (this is your new middle section). Take the section of hair on the right side and go under the middle section (this is your new middle section).

3. Take a small section of hair from the right, above the braid, add it to the right-hand section, and go under into the middle.

4. Alternating right to left, continue the lace-braid technique. Only add hair from the right as you work down the side of the head.

5. When you reach your ear, continue with a three-strand braid (see page 51) and secure with a hair elastic. With the curling iron, curl the hair in the middle of the hair section (see beach waves, page 24).

TIP

Make sure your hair is well brushed for this style. You want it to hang neatly down out of the braid, so you don't want any tangles getting in the way.

39. ASYMMETRIC CORNROW

BEST FOR

 THICK

CURLY

WAVY

FRIZZY

The cornrow asymmetric style is for the rocker chick and is great to wear for any concert or festival. This style includes a side Dutch braid, giving the appearance that your hair is shorter on one side, with loose waves to soften the look. If you can already do a Dutch braid, this style is easy to achieve. It works perfectly for the girl who has thick hair and wants to tuck some of the bulk away from her face in a braid. I also recommend this style for anyone who has wavy hair. The cornrow will blend beautifully into your waves. It's an edgy look and can also look fantastic with frizzy hair too, as the cornrow helps tame wild or voluminous hair. If your hair isn't wavy or curly, refer to the beach waves tutorial (see page 24) to make your hair wavy before you start.

▶ **SEE ALSO**
Lace braid with waves, page 64

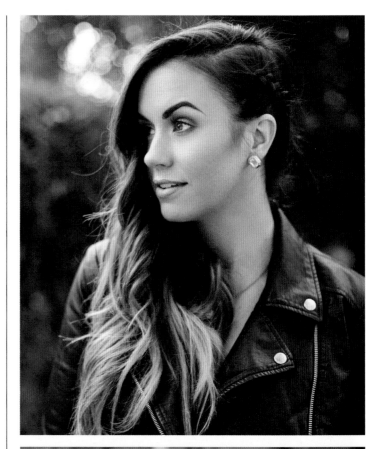

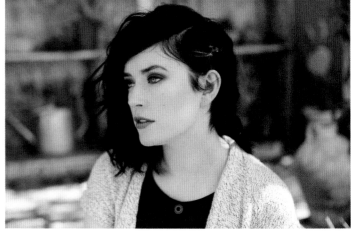

HOW TO DO IT

WHAT YOU NEED

- Comb
- Hair clip
- Hair elastic
- Medium-hold hairspray

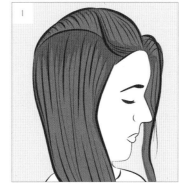

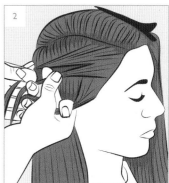

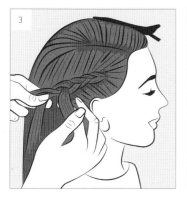

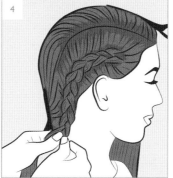

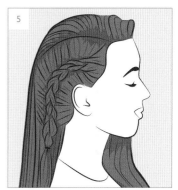

1. Create a deep side part on the desired side by going as far over as the arch of your brow line. From that parting, create a large C-like section from the hairline down to the side of the nape of your neck, about an inch away from the middle of the back of your neck. Clip back the hair above the C-like section.

2. Start to make a Dutch braid (see page 90) inside the C-like section going from your hairline back to the nape of the neck, down the center of your section.

3. As you work toward the back of your neck, incorporate hair into your braid from both sides, keeping the braid central.

4. When you reach the nape, secure the braid with a hair elastic.

5. Let the ends of the Dutch braid blend in with the rest of your hair. Finish off the look by using a medium-hold hairspray.

TIP

If your hair doesn't reach the back of your neck, stop the braid where your hair ends and bobby pin it into place. Feel free to get creative and use a decorative bobby pin or criss cross your bobby pins.

CHAPTER 3
SPORTY

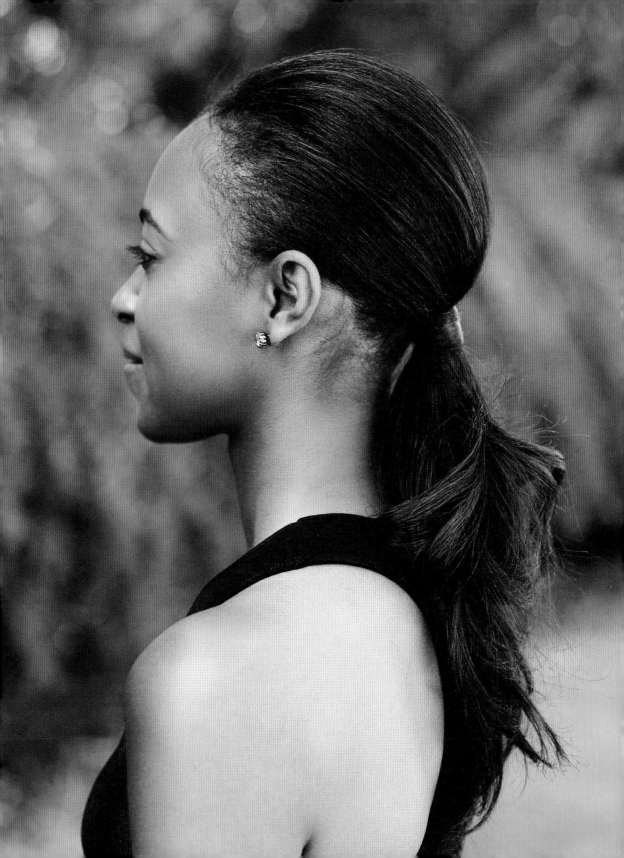

40. PIGTAILS

BEST FOR

 WAVY

 FRIZZY

Pigtails don't have to be just for kids—anyone can wear this hairstyle. This look is usually worn casually and is great for the beach or gym. I love this look on slightly wavy hair, which gives some style to the look and helps make it look more adult. I also recommend pigtails for anyone who has a bit of chemical texture or frizz to their hair from coloring; this prevents the style from looking silky and "young." This style will work best if your hair is at least collarbone length —you need enough hair to come out of the pigtails to make it dramatic.

▶ **SEE ALSO**
Low pony, page 76

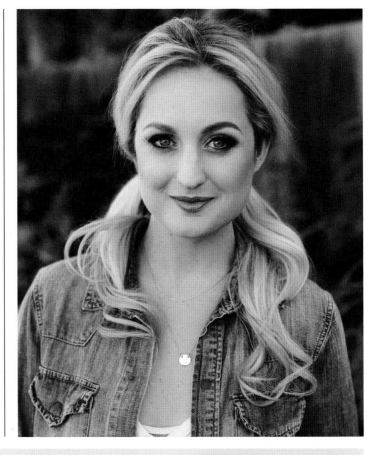

41. BRAIDED PIGTAILS

You can make your pigtails look more interesting by simply adding a few braids into the style. You need really long hair for this style because once you do your braid, you will lose a lot of the length. Divide your hair in half as in the pigtail tutorial, but add a simple three-strand braid (see page 51) into the hair for a few inches and secure the ends with a hair elastic to hold it into place. Finish off the look with a flexible-hold hairspray.

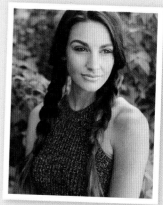

HOW TO DO IT

WHAT YOU NEED

- Comb
- Hair elastics
- Bobby pins
- Flexible-hold hairspray

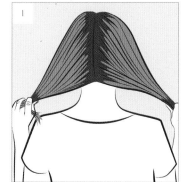

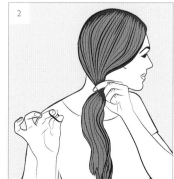

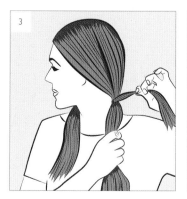

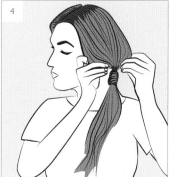

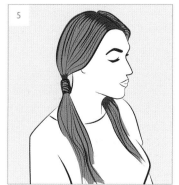

1. Split your hair in half from the center of your hairline all the way to the nape of your neck.

2. Comb all of the hair from the right side of the split and gather it down toward the area right behind your ear. Secure it with a hair elastic, making sure it is fairly tight. Repeat on the other side.

3. To dress up your pigtails, take a small section of hair from underneath the ponytail and wrap it securely around the hair elastic. Use a bobby pin to secure it in place under your ponytail.

4. Gently pull on the hair above the pigtails so it is not so snug to the head—this also gives it a little bit more body.

5. Finish off the look by spraying with a flexible-hold hairspray.

TIP

If your hair doesn't have wave to it or isn't chemically textured, blow dry a texturizer in your hair from roots to ends, and throw in some beach waves before getting started (see page 24).

42. MESSY SIDE PONY

BEST FOR

☰ FINE

Sometimes messy can look more chic than sleek, and in my opinion, a good messy side pony is the only way to do a low pony. This look is ideal if your hair is fine with layers, and it's best on second-day hair. The layers will give your hair volume, while slightly dirty hair, with its natural separation and texture, creates a disheveled look. This style looks best on hair that is mid-length to long. If you don't have second-day hair and crave this style, throw in a little spray wax in your hair before getting started to aid separation.

▶ **SEE ALSO**
Low pony, page 76

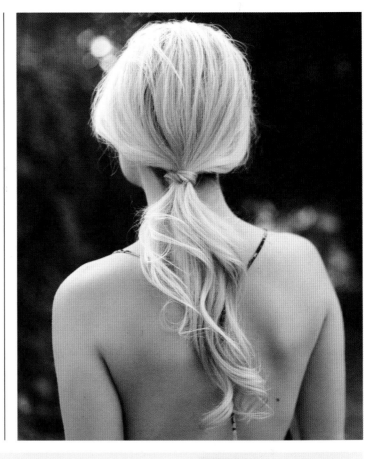

43. MESSY SIDE PONY WITH FLORAL HEADBAND

You can change the whole look of your messy side pony by leaving a few pieces of hair out around the face and curling them as well as adding a few curls to the hair in your ponytail to create more fullness. This look works best with curly hair or pre-curled hair (see natural curly hair, page 28). Then you can adorn your hair with a gorgeous floral headpiece and it will change up the look completely.

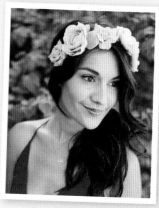

HOW TO DO IT

WHAT YOU NEED

- Comb
- Hair powder or dry shampoo (optional)
- Hair elastic
- Bobby pin
- Flexible-hold hairspray

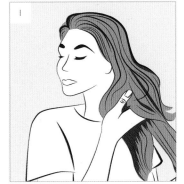
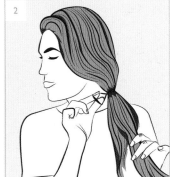
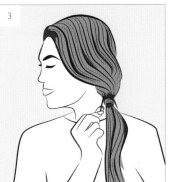
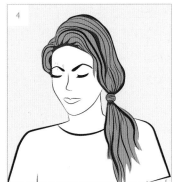

1. Start with 100 percent dry hair. Gather your hair to the desired side. Lightly tease it upward so that it creates a lot of bulk and gives your hair a slight messy texture. If your hair is really silky, you can grunge up the texture by adding a hair powder or dry shampoo. This will make the hair appear thicker and create grip to hold it in place.

2. Lightly gather the hair to just below the ear and secure it in place with a hair elastic. Don't take out too much of your light teasing.

3. To add a little flair to your simple pony, wind hair around your ponytail so that you hide the hair elastic. You can do this by taking a ½-in (1.3-cm) section of hair from underneath the hair left out of your ponytail, wrapping it around your hair elastic, and securing it into your ponytail with a bobby pin.

4. Use a flexible-hold hairspray to give hold but allow some movement.

TIP

If your hair is fine or thick and doesn't have much volume, try curling it with flexible-hold hairspray before putting it in your side ponytail.

44. HIGH PONYTAIL

BEST FOR

 STRAIGHT

▦ THICK

The high ponytail is flattering for most face shapes and it's easy to do. When the ponytail is in place on the high crown area, it helps lift the face. This hairstyle is ideal for girls with naturally straight, thick hair and a silky texture. When the hair is already silky, it really helps take this high ponytail to the next level and make it ultra chic. If your hair isn't naturally silky and straight, I recommend adding a gloss serum from roots to ends and blow drying it straight prior to getting started.

▶ **SEE ALSO**
Fishtail pony,
page 82

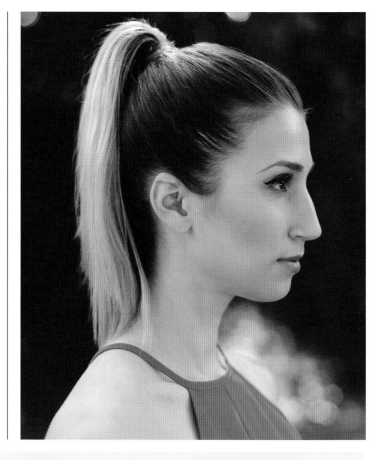

45. HALF PONYTAIL

The half pony is a very casual style and works well for mid-length hair. It's great if your hair is extremely thick because it allows you to wear your hair down but you have most of it pulled back and out of your face. You can achieve a half ponytail by sectioning out the top half of your hair from ear to ear, combing it back, gathering this section of hair into a ponytail, and securing it with a hair elastic. To dress up your pony, take a small section of hair from underneath the ponytail and wrap it around the hair elastic to cover it up. Finish off with a medium-hold hairspray.

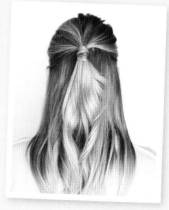

HOW TO DO IT

WHAT YOU NEED

- Comb
- 1 or 2 hair elastics
- Bobby pins
- Light hairspray (optional)

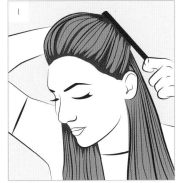

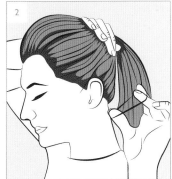

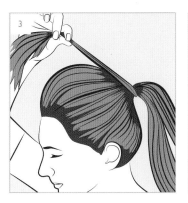

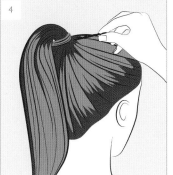

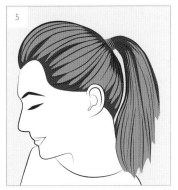

1. Comb all of your hair toward the crown of the head. Gather all of your hair with one hand while brushing it toward the crown.

2. Secure your hair at the high crown area with a hair elastic. If your hair is thick, use two hair elastics.

3. Take a small section of hair from the ponytail and wrap it around the hair elastic.

4. Secure the hair you wrapped around the ponytail with a bobby pin underneath. This will hide the elastic and create a more finished look.

5. If you have any unwanted flyaways around your face or around your ponytail, use a light hairspray and spray in the direction of the crown while lightly smoothing out your hair with your fingers. This will give your ponytail a chic look.

TIP

If your ponytail starts to look droopy, add a bobby pin or two in the middle of the hair elastic. This will allow the pony to stick out from the base, giving it more bounce.

46. LOW PONY

BEST FOR

 THICK

 FRIZZY

The low pony is one of those simple classic styles that can be worn in a number of ways from sporty to chic. This look is a great option for girls who have extremely thick hair. Thick hair can be very heavy and will usually fall flat anyway, so if it's low in the first place you can prevent this happening and achieve a really gorgeous look. It's also great for frizzy hair, as keeping the pony low helps keep unruly hair out of the way and under control. I also love it on mid-length to long hair—the length adds drama to the pony.

▶ **SEE ALSO**
High ponytail, page 74

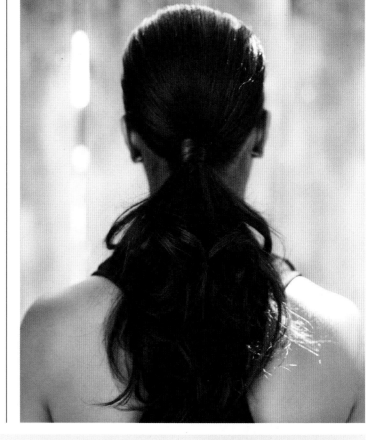

47. FRENCH BACK PONY

This style is perfect for anyone with heavy, limp hair that just won't hold in a ponytail. You can easily reduce bulk and jazz up your thick locks by adding a small French braid to your pony. Divide a small section of hair at the front of your head into three parts and create a French braid (see page 80). Continue the French braid technique for a few inches and then switch to a basic three-strand braid (see page 51). Secure the ends with a hair elastic, then pull all of your hair into a ponytail.

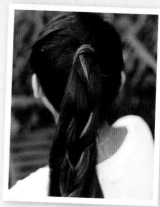

HOW TO DO IT

WHAT YOU NEED

- Hairbrush
- Hair elastic
- Bobby pin
- Medium-hold hairspray

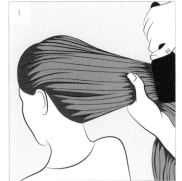
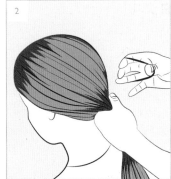
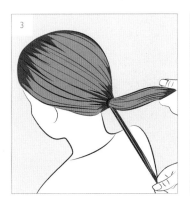
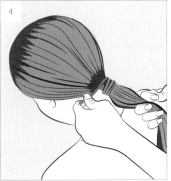
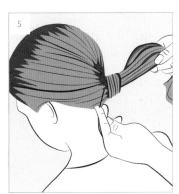

1. Brush all your hair back toward the nape of the neck.
2. Gather all of the hair together and secure tightly with a hair elastic to create your low ponytail.
3. Take a small piece of hair from underneath the ponytail.
4. Wrap the small section of hair around the base of the ponytail.
5. Take the end of this section of hair and thread it through a bobby pin and pin it into the base of the ponytail. Finish off this look with a medium-hold hairspray.

TIP

If you crave a long low pony but your hair is on the shorter side, add some hair wefts (or extensions) after you have secured your pony and blend them in by wrapping pieces of hair over the ponytail.

48. DUTCH BRAID IN PONY

BEST FOR

≡ FINE
≡ FLAT

Sometimes you want to add a little spice to your ponytail, especially when your hair is fine or flat and you can't achieve a full ponytail look. The Dutch braid in pony is perfect for this. The style also looks great when your hair is really long with minimal layers, which creates a dramatic ponytail. It's a fabulous style to wear to a ball game or an outdoor event.

▶ **SEE ALSO**
Fishtail pony, page 82

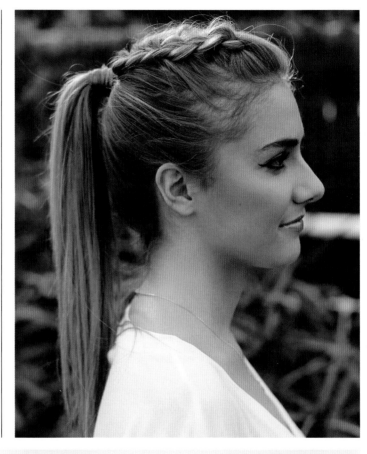

49. VIKING BRAID

Transform your Dutch braid pony to a statement braided style by turning it into a Viking braid. This style works best on extremely long hair with minimal layers. To achieve this style, use the Dutch braid technique as in the above tutorial but continue to braid your hair all the way to the ends and secure with a hair elastic. Then aggressively "pancake" your braid by pulling it out for fullness and pull all of your hair into a ponytail. If you're feeling extra sassy, try making a braid on each side for this hairstyle.

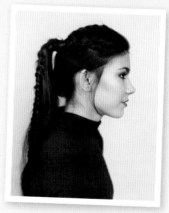

HOW TO DO IT

WHAT YOU NEED

 PARTNER

- Hair elastics
- Comb
- Medium-hold hairspray

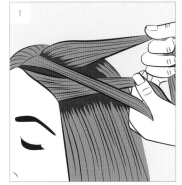

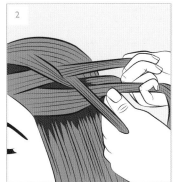

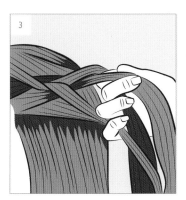

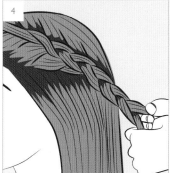

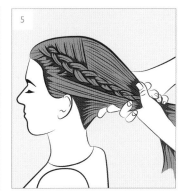

1. Starting at the part of your hair, divide a section of hair into three small, even sections. Take the small piece of hair closest to the part and cross it under into the middle section. Then take the small section of hair from around the hairline and go under into the middle section.

2. Now add hair into your braid as you work the hair back. Do this by working from right to left, adding a small piece of hair to each small section on the outside of the braid as you go. First, add a piece of hair from the right.

3. Add a small piece of hair from the left.

4. Continue for a few inches back around your hairline and then work a three-strand braid (see page 51). Secure the ends with a hair elastic.

5. Gather all of the hair, with your Dutch braid, toward the crown area, and make a ponytail. Secure with a hair elastic and hairspray to finish.

TIP

If your hair is really thick and you want to achieve this look, simply don't pull the braid out too much, otherwise the fuller Dutch braid will overshadow your ponytail.

50. FRENCH BRAID

BEST FOR

 THICK

 FRIZZY

This classic has made a big comeback now that braids are all the rage. The French braid hairstyle can be worn on every woman no matter what her age and still look stylish. The simple French braid hairstyle works well with long hair with minimal layers. This style looks most dramatic when you have a bit of hair color contrast or highlights to show the elegance of the woven pieces. You can wear this hairstyle casually for an active day or to go shopping. It's also a really good way of taming frizzy hair if you're on the go or at the gym.

▶ **SEE ALSO**
Dutch braid, page 90

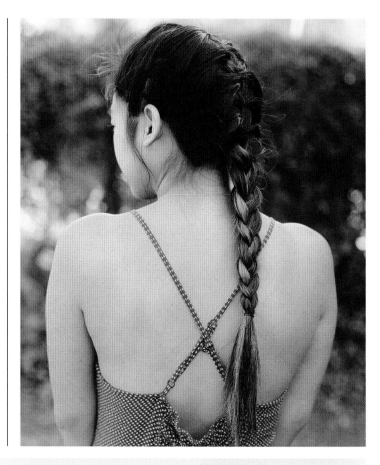

51. SIDE FRENCH BRAID

Easily change up your French braid look by creating a side French braid. This style is good for ladies with long hair, and it works especially well on hair that is dirty because your natural oils allow the hair to look smooth and stay in place. Instead of creating your French braid from your hairline to the nape of your neck, start from your hairline and work your way down toward your ear then to your neck. Finish off with a three-strand braid to the end (see page 51) and secure with a hair elastic.

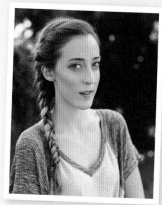

HOW TO DO IT

WHAT YOU NEED

 PARTNER

- Brush
- Hair elastics
- Medium-hold hairspray

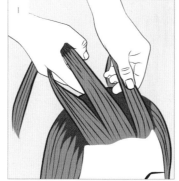

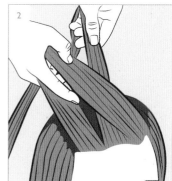

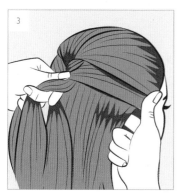

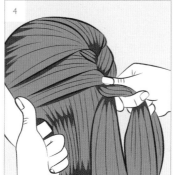

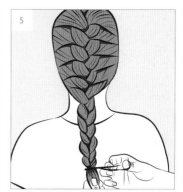

1. Take a small half-moon section at the top of your head starting at the hairline, and divide it into three clean and equal strands. Hold two of the strands in one hand and the third in the other hand.

2. Take the strand of hair from the left and cross it up and over into the center. Cross the right strand up and over into the center.

3. Incorporate new hair by grabbing another strand of hair from the loose section of hair on the same side. Include it in your strand and cross it up and over into the center.

4. Repeat this same technique on the opposite side by incorporating hair on the right side and cross over to the center. Continue down to your ears and neck.

5. When you run out of hair to French braid, continue doing a simple three-strand braid technique (see page 51). When you get to the ends, secure the braid with a hair elastic. Use medium-hold hairspray to hold the braid in place.

TIP

If you want your braid to be thicker, use a little bit of hairspray all over your hair, and lightly tug on each section of hair to make it appear fuller, but be careful not to pull it out completely.

52. FISHTAIL PONY

BEST FOR

 THICK

 STRAIGHT

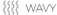 WAVY

The fishtail pony is fun, flirty, and functional. This look is simple but the fishtail packs a lot of punch. This style is a fishtail braid and pony combined and can be worn in several ways—make it casual or dress it up. This look works best on long, straight, quite thick hair, and it makes a great second-day hairstyle. This fishtail pony is useful for keeping your hair out of your face for outdoor activities or an exercise class.

▶ **SEE ALSO**
Dutch braid in pony, page 78

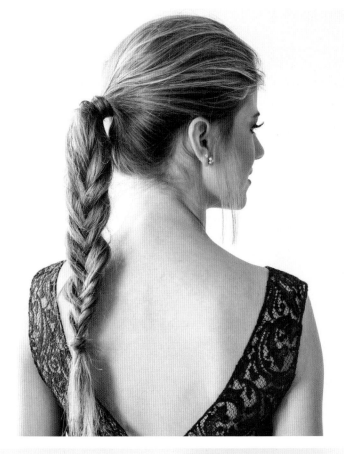

53. BRAIDED PONY

If you don't want to wear a fishtail pony, you can achieve a pony that's just as cool by doing the braided pony style. This style is sophisticated yet works for sporty girls. It works particularly well with medium to thick long hair, and hair that has a bit of chemical texture, which will prevent the braid from falling flat. Instead of doing a fishtail braid inside your pony, do a simple three-strand braid (see page 51) and secure with a hair elastic.

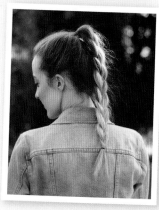

HOW TO DO IT

WHAT YOU NEED

 PARTNER

- Hair elastic
- Bobby pins
- Comb
- 2 hair clips
- Flexible-hold hairspray

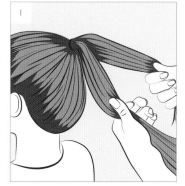

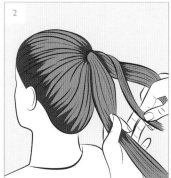

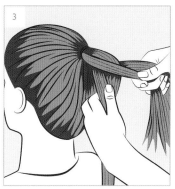

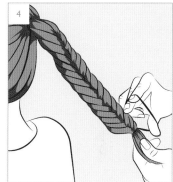

1. Gather the hair on top of your head to create a high pony at the crown area, and secure it with a hair elastic. Divide the hair inside the ponytail into two equal sections.

2. Take a small section of hair from the outside of the right section, and bring that section up and over into the left section. That piece is now a part of the left section.

3. Repeat on the opposite side, taking a small section of hair from the left section and crossing over to the right section.

4. Continue the fishtail-braid pattern until you get to the ends of the hair and secure them with a hair elastic. Finish off the look with a flexible-hold hairspray.

TIP

If you want your braid to be bigger and fuller, try gently tugging on each fishtail strand to plump it up.

54. WOVEN PONY

BEST FOR

 CURLY

 THICK

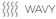 WAVY

The woven ponytail dresses up the regular pony—you create a low pony and weave pieces across it for a unique effect. It's just casual enough for hanging out with girlfriends or weekend errands or you can add a hair embellishment and wear it for a formal occasion. This hairstyle looks best on hair that has a wavy to curly hair texture. I also love it on thick hair because the hair left out of the pony will look full. It's also great if you have some layers so that some strands will naturally fall out, giving a really romantic, undone finish.

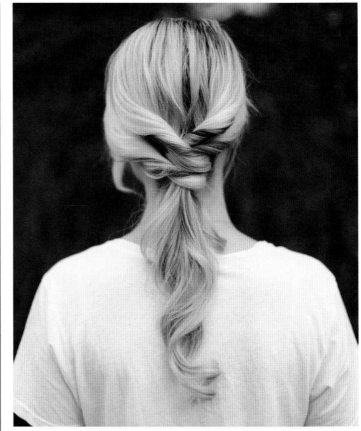

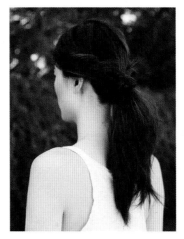

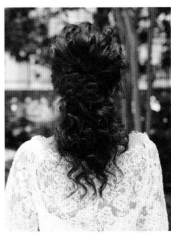

▶ **SEE ALSO**
Topsy-tail pony, page 30

HOW TO DO IT

WHAT YOU NEED

- 2 hair clips
- Hair elastic
- Bobby pins
- Comb
- Medium-hold hairspray

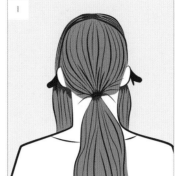

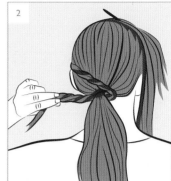

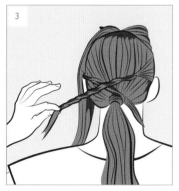

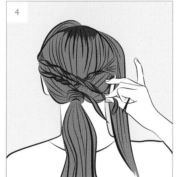

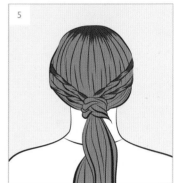

1. Section out both sides of the hair in front of the ears and clip back.

2. Create a low pony at the nape of neck and secure it with a hair elastic.

3. Drop out the sections in front. Take a 1–2-in (2.5–5-cm) section above the left ear and clip back the rest. Twist back, going toward the ponytail on the other side. If your hair is really long, wrap the ends around your ponytail. Secure the end of the twist with bobby pins.

4. Repeat this technique on the right side. Always work left to right so that the twists lie on top of each other. Then drop the next section on your left. (If your hair is really thick you may need to do more than two twists on each side.)

5. Twist back your remaining hair, drape it across to the opposite side of your ponytail, and bobby pin into place. Repeat on the right side. Finish off by using a medium-hold hairspray.

TIP

To make this look a bit more fancy, try curling the hair beforehand, which will create more body as well as a pretty curl to the hair.

55. LOW CHIC PONYTAIL

BEST FOR

 STRAIGHT

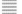 FLAT

The low chic ponytail is truly versatile and will look good no matter what you're doing and where you're going. I recommend this style for hair that is naturally straight or flat with a soft, silky texture and minimal layers. This allows you to create a clean and tidy look with no strands out of place. It's also good for women with prominent cheekbones because it will really help bring out your facial features. If you don't have straight hair and you would love to achieve this look, follow the straight hair tutorial (see page 42) before you start.

▶ **SEE ALSO**
Low pony, page 76

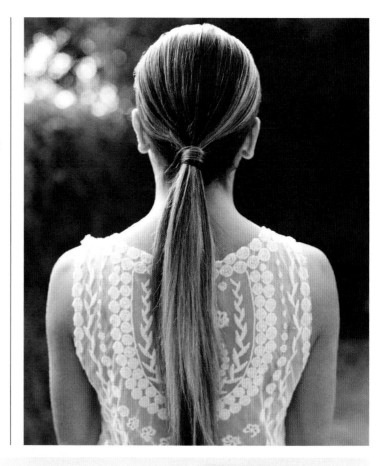

56. SIDE CHIC PONYTAIL

A low chic ponytail can easily be turned into a chic side pony and you get a totally different look. It looks especially gorgeous on ladies who have extremely long hair with few layers. I love this look on dirty hair because the natural oils help tame flyaways. You can achieve this look by combing the hair to the side where you want to position your side pony and securing the pony with a hair elastic. Finish off the look by using a shine spray for ultra sleekness.

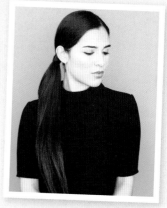

HOW TO DO IT

WHAT YOU NEED

- Hair clip
- Silkening creme
- Flat brush
- Hair elastic
- Firm-hold hairspray

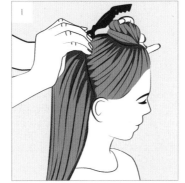

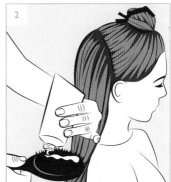

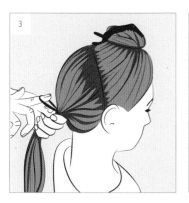

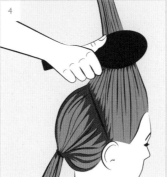

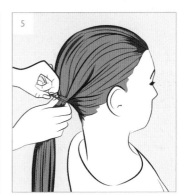

1. Start with pre-straightened hair that is 100 percent dry. Divide the hair into two sections around the ear area from side to side. Clip back the front section.

2. Apply the silkening creme onto a flat brush, and brush the product into your hair toward the nape of your neck as you gather the hair together.

3. Create a tight low ponytail and secure it with a hair elastic.

4. Release the front section of hair. To create the same sleekness as the bottom pony, apply some silkening creme on your brush and brush your hair toward the nape of your neck as you did in Step 2.

5. Once the hair is sleek to the head, gather the top section with the first ponytail and secure with an elastic, then wrap a small section of hair around the elastic and pin. Finish with a firm-hold hairspray.

TIP

If you end up with a lot of lumps and bumps in your ponytail, the trick is to take the end of a weaving comb, put it in your hair at the hairline and gently move toward your low pony area to remove the bumps.

57. UPSIDE-DOWN FRENCH BACK BUN

BEST FOR

 THICK

 WAVY

@ CURLY

The upside-down French back bun is a great alternative to a top knot and adds some spice to your hairdo. This works best on hair that is at least mid-length so you have enough hair to braid with plenty left over for the bun. This look works well on thick hair that is dirty and is best for wavy to curly hair; the texture will create volume in your bun.

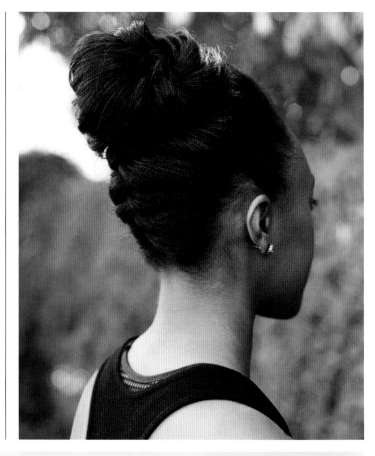

▶ **SEE ALSO**
High fishtail bun, page 56

58. UPSIDE-DOWN FRENCH BACK PONY

If having all of your hair in a bun isn't your thing, try an upside-down French back pony, where the hair is left out in a ponytail when your braid reaches the top of your crown. For this style you need long hair so you have enough hair left out of your ponytail. I also recommend this style on wavy hair so it makes the pony look dressed up. If you don't have waves, just throw a few soft curls in your hair (see page 28) for a beautiful wavy texture. For details of how to do a French braid, see page 80.

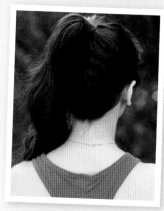

HOW TO DO IT

WHAT YOU NEED

 PARTNER

- Brush
- Hair clip
- 2 hair elastics
- Bobby pins
- Lightweight hairspray

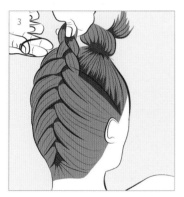

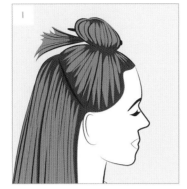

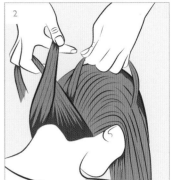

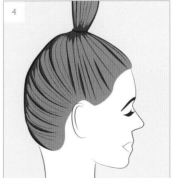

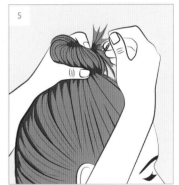

1. Section off the front section from ear to ear across the crown area and clip back for later.

2. Flip your head upside down and start a normal French braid technique by taking a small section of hair at the nape of your neck and dividing it into three equal sections. See French braid (page 80) for details.

3. Start to connect hair from the sides as you work from the nape to your crown area. Secure the base of your braid to the scalp with a hair elastic.

4. Drop the hair out of your clipped-back section, add it to your hair outside the braided pony and secure with a hair elastic.

5. Wrap all the hair around the pony to make a bun and secure with bobby pins. Finish off this look with a lightweight hairspray.

TIP

Don't feel left out if your hair is on the shorter side. You can easily throw in some extensions for extra length and wrap them into a fun bun. No one will ever know.

59. DUTCH BRAID

BEST FOR

 FINE

FLAT

A French braid might be fun but the Dutch braid has a little more drama—it is done underhanded so the braid itself will show inside out. You need long hair for this style. It works especially well for ladies who have hair that is flat or on the finer side and want to make it look fuller. You can simply pull the braid out a little at the end to instantly create a fuller appearance. Dutch braids also work well on chemically textured hair, which will stay in place once pulled out. If you don't have that type of texture, throw a salt spray in your hair to add some grit and create hold.

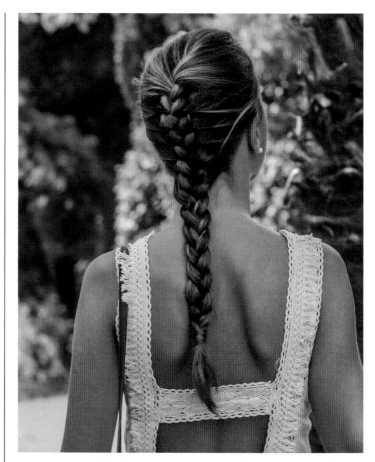

▶ **SEE ALSO**
French braid,
page 80

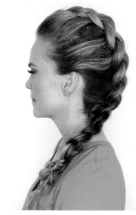

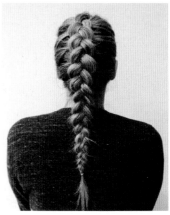

HOW TO DO IT

WHAT YOU NEED

 PARTNER

- Brush
- Hair elastics

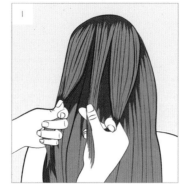

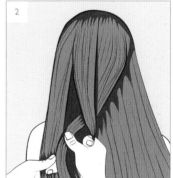

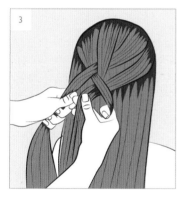

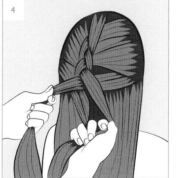

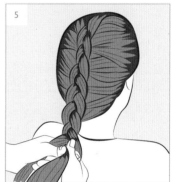

1. Position your fingers up and the back of your hands down so you always braid your hair underhanded. Take a half-moon section from the front of the hairline and divide your hair into three equal sections.

2. Take the section on your right and go under the middle section into the middle. Repeat on the opposite side, taking your left section and going under into the middle section. This is your new middle section.

3. Start adding hair into your braid as you work from the hairline down to the nape of your neck. Take a small piece of hair from the right side of your hairline back to your braid and take that whole section under into the middle of the braid. Repeat on the other side.

4. Continue to work this pattern and add hair to your Dutch braid, working the sections right to left. Continue to the nape of the neck.

5. Do a three-strand braid (see page 51); secure with an elastic.

TIP

To create more volume, blow dry a volumizing product in your hair before you start. Dry it from underneath, pulling up at the roots. This will give you a fuller Dutch-braid look.

CHAPTER 4
DRESS UP

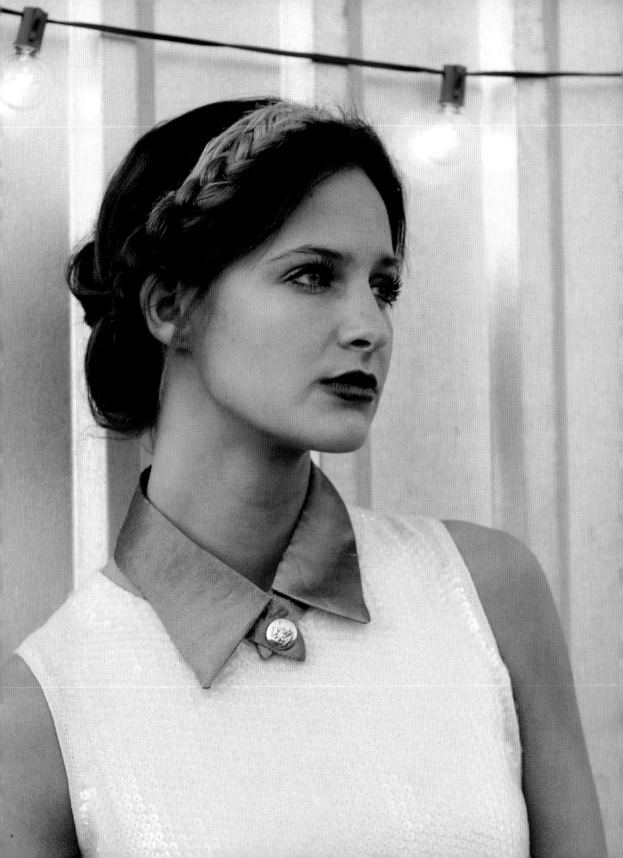

60. BOUFFANT BUN

BEST FOR

 THICK

 FRIZZY

If you have thick, frizzy hair and you want to make the best of your own natural texture, this is the ideal dressy look for you. The bouffant bun is a bit bigger than a standard top knot but is just as sassy and it's perfect if your hair is really thick with frizz. You also need long hair for this look because it helps add to the height of the bun. If you don't have frizzy hair, try adding texture to your hair by using a dry shampoo and roughing up the cuticle by teasing your hair aggressively. You're sure to be the talk of the party with this do.

▶ **SEE ALSO**
Sock bun, page 58

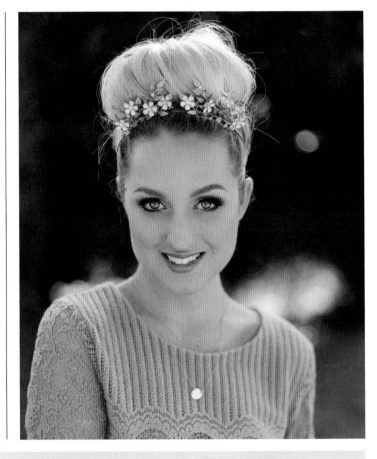

61. BOUFFANT BUN WITH BRAID

Want to create a little more interest in your bouffant bun? Try accenting it with a beautiful braid. I love this style on extremely long hair, which allows you to create a really big bun and braid. All you have to do is leave a small section of hair out of your ponytail before creating your bouffant bun. Once you've made the bun, braid that section. Wrap your braid across the bun and bobby pin it into place.

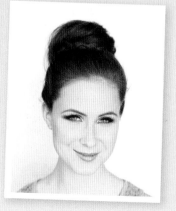

HOW TO DO IT

WHAT YOU NEED

- Brush
- Hair elastic or clip
- Bobby pins
- Firm-hold hairspray

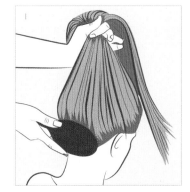

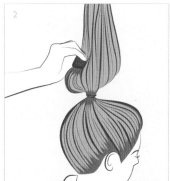

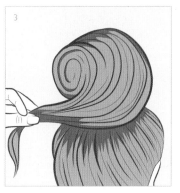

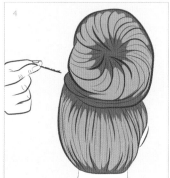

1. Create a high ponytail by brushing your hair all the way up to the crown of the head and securing the hair in a hair elastic or clip.

2. Add bulk to your pony by aggressively teasing your hair at the base. If your hair is silky and doesn't hold backcombing very well, use some hairspray first.

3. Wrap your teased ponytail around the base of your ponytail, making sure you do not wrap it too tightly because you want your bouffant to have a lot of bulk.

4. Secure your bouffant bun by adding a few bobby pins toward the base of your ponytail. Finish off this look by using a firm-hold hairspray.

TIP

If you love this look but don't have the length or thickness, you can easily fake it by adding a few clip-in extensions at the ponytail area and gently teasing them before you start.

62. HEADBAND TWIST AND TUCK

BEST FOR

 WAVY

Who doesn't love a good updo that looks complicated but takes minutes? I love this look on ladies with mid-length hair so the hairstyle doesn't look too bulky. It also works well with slightly wavy hair—the waves help your hair stay around the headband. It looks terrific on hair that has some layers around the face, as wisps of hair slip out creating a soft look. You can go for a bohemian or classic feel depending on the type of headband you choose. Make the look a little more boho by creating beach waves in your hair and throwing in a headscarf.

▶ **SEE ALSO**
Headband braid,
page 34

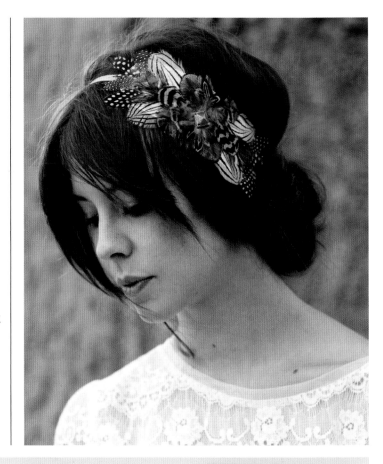

63. GIBSON TUCK

If you don't have a headband for the twist and tuck, you can try the Gibson tuck. This is a great style for ladies who have chemically textured hair or as a second-day do. For this look, use a similar technique as the twist and tuck but twist your hair inward on each side until it creates a roll working toward the back of your head. Continue until your hair is fully twisted, and tuck the ends inside your roll. Secure the hair into place with bobby pins. Finish off this look with a medium-hold hairspray.

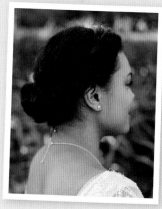

HOW TO DO IT

WHAT YOU NEED

- Headband that goes all around the head
- Medium-hold hairspray

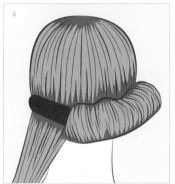

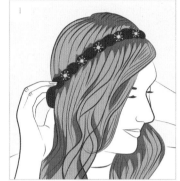

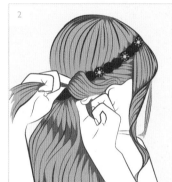

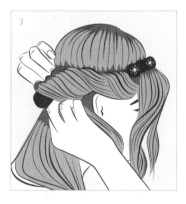

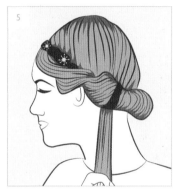

1. Start with 100 percent dry hair. If you want more curl or texture, feel free to curl your hair before attempting this hairstyle. Then put on your headband.

2. Starting on the right side of your head, take a section of hair and wrap it up and over the rolled band, pulling the ends through the other side of the band.

3. Take the same section of hair, include a new section as well, and wrap up and over the rolled band again.

4. Repeat this technique until you get to the middle of the back of your head.

5. Repeat the same technique on the other side. Use a medium-hold hairspray to finish.

TIP

Feel free to get creative and add extra interest to your headband style by braiding a few sections before rolling them into your headband.

64. MILKMAID BRAID

BEST FOR

~~~~ WAVY

|||||| STRAIGHT

The milkmaid braid is a simple, beautiful everyday style. This delicate style has been around for ages and has stood the test of time because it is still very popular to this day! This style works well with straight or wavy hair so that you can see the definition in the braid and it's perfect if you have extremely long hair—the braid has to reach the other side of the head to achieve the true milkmaid effect. Even beginner braiders can create this style. It simply involves braiding each side of the hair and draping the braids over the top of the head.

▶ **SEE ALSO**
   Headband braid,
   page 34

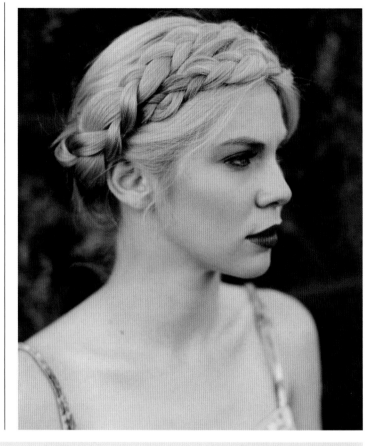

65. FISHTAIL MILKMAID BRAID

Loving this style but want to take it to the next level? Go for fishtail braids instead of regular three-strand braids to jazz up your milkmaid braid. It works best if you have straight, long hair—you need plenty of length for fishtail braids. Simply create two fishtail braids instead of the standard braid (see page 38). Wrap the braids over one another and bobby pin them into place.

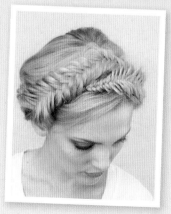

HOW TO DO IT

WHAT YOU NEED

- Brush
- Hair elastics
- Bobby pins

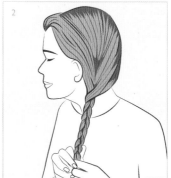

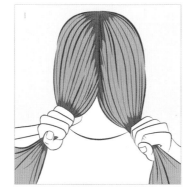

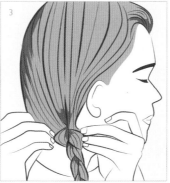

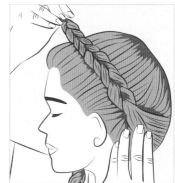

1. Start with dry hair. Divide the hair in half from the middle of the hairline down to the nape of the neck.

2. Split one side into three sections and apply a simple three-strand braid technique (see page 51). Continue this technique until you have no more hair to work with and secure the ends with a hair elastic.

3. Repeat the same technique on the other side. Then tug the sides of the braids to plump them out and add volume.

4. Once both sections have been braided, wrap the right braid across the front of your hairline and bobby pin the ends into the scalp. Take the left braid and wrap it over to the right side, directly behind the first braid, and secure it with bobby pins.

TIP

For a whimsical feel to your braid, apply a lightweight hairspray and massage the hair with your palms for softness and to create little wispy bits.

66. FLOWER BUN

BEST FOR

 THICK

 FLAT

The flower bun is an elegant hairstyle that gives the look of simplicity from the front and has added interest from the back. This low-volume look works beautifully on ladies who have thicker hair that tends to fall flat. It looks especially lovely on wavy hair, which makes the style look bohemian and carefree. You could easily wear this look to a bridal shower or for a casual stroll through the park. If your hair isn't wavy, feel free to throw in some waves before you get started.

▶ **SEE ALSO**
Ponytail bow, page 104

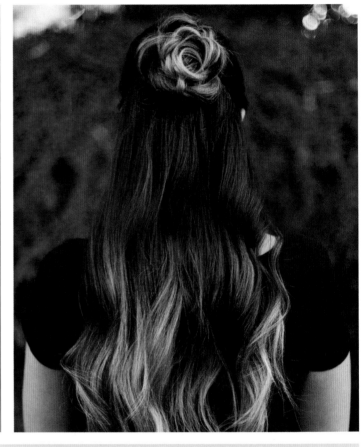

67. CRISS-CROSS FLOWER BUN UPDO

You can easily step up your flower bun a notch by creating a beautiful updo. This look will suit you if you have extremely long, medium-thick hair with a bit of chemical texture. Divide your hair in half in the back and use the fishtail braid technique (see page 38). Continue this technique until you get to a few inches below the crown, secure the hair into a ponytail, and continue with the flower-bun technique as in the main tutorial.

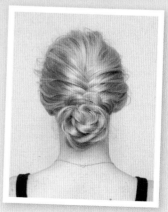

HOW TO DO IT

WHAT YOU NEED

- Comb
- Hair elastics
- Bobby pins
- Medium-hold hairspray

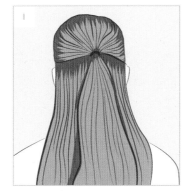

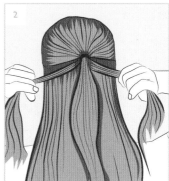

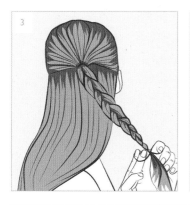

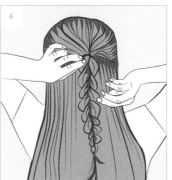

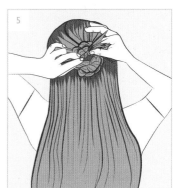

1. Start with dry hair. If your hair is dirty, add some dry shampoo to help soak up any excess oils. Divide your hair in half across the back of your head from ear to ear and gather the hair together. Secure with a hair elastic.

2. Divide the hair in the band into three even sections.

3. Make a simple three-strand braid (see page 51) until you get to the ends and secure it with a hair elastic.

4. Pull on the right side of the braid gently to create a "pancake" braiding effect. This will plump up the side of the braid that will form the outside of the flower bun.

5. Create a bun, with the side of the braid that you pancaked on the outer side, and secure in place with bobby pins. Use a medium-hold hairspray to finish.

TIP

If your hair is silky and won't pull out very well, then use hairspray on the braid before pulling the right side out. This will allow it to have a bit of texture and the braid will be sturdier.

68. HALF-UP BOUFFANT

BEST FOR

 STRAIGHT

FLAT

WAVY

The half-up bouffant style is perfect for girls whose hair generally falls flat, because it creates volume and fullness. It's good for mid-length to long hair and works well if you like to wear some of your hair down. This style is lovely with straight to wavy hair, which allows your bouffant to be smooth and full but not overly frizzy. The half-up bouffant is smart and glamourous enough for any business event or formal social occasion.

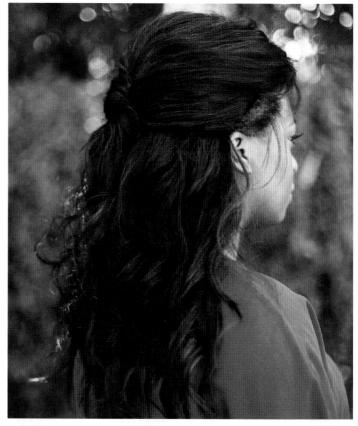

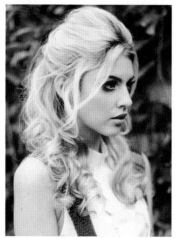

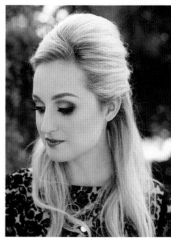

▶ **SEE ALSO**
Bouffant bun, page 94

HOW TO DO IT

WHAT YOU NEED

 PARTNER

- Comb
- Bobby pins
- Medium-hold hairspray

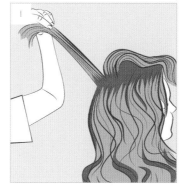

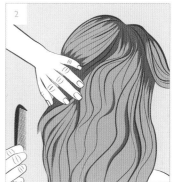

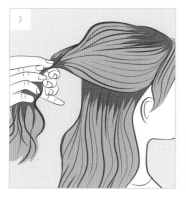

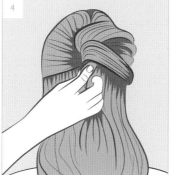

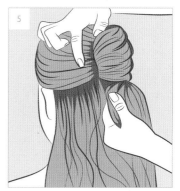

1. Start with dry hair. Begin at the crown of your head. Take a horizontal section of hair and lightly tease the root area. Continue in the same way, working up to a couple of inches away from your hairline.

2. Part your hair on the desired side and gently pull it back toward the back of the bottom of your crown.

3. Gather the whole top section of hair that you teased back, and twist it.

4. Push the twist up against the scalp. By doing this, you are not only creating a decorative style, but you are also helping the hair stay into place and maintaining the volume.

5. Pull on each side of the hair at the roots of the twisted section to create an even, rounded shape. Bobby pin the twist into place at the base. If your hair is extremely thick, you might need to use several pins. Finish off the look with a medium-hold hairspray.

TIP

For extra volume at the roots that will hold all day, try using a dry shampoo or a style dust at the roots before you tease the hair.

69. PONYTAIL BOW

BEST FOR

 THICK

 WAVY

The ponytail bow is fun, flirty, and girly. It might look plain at first but once people take a good look at the back they will be pleasantly surprised by this cute do. This look works best for thick hair, which allows you to create a full ponytail bow. It also suits ladies with a silky hair texture so the definition in the bow can be clearly seen. This hairstyle works best for formal affairs, such as weddings, showers, and dances. If your hair is really curly and you want to sport this style, I recommend straightening it first so that the bow shape holds and stands out.

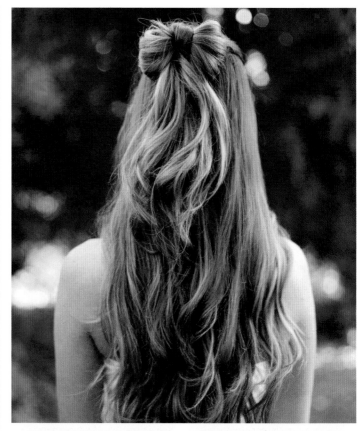

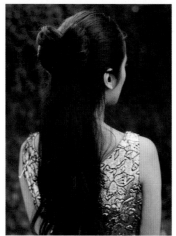

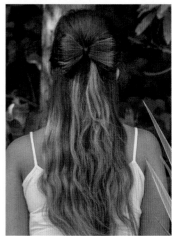

▶ **SEE ALSO**
Flower bun, page 100

HOW TO DO IT

WHAT YOU NEED

- Comb or brush
- Hair elastic
- Hair clip
- A few bobby pins

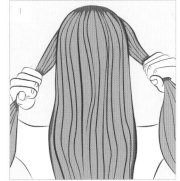

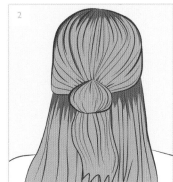

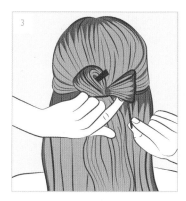

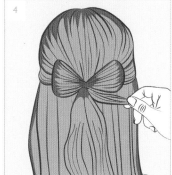

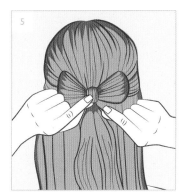

1. Take one small section of hair from each side of your head—the bigger the sections, the bigger the bow.

2. Tie the two sections together with a hair elastic to create a half ponytail. Don't pull the ends all the way through the elastic so that you create a loop (see low looped pony, page 14).

3. Split the loop in half to create two smaller loops and clip one loop aside. Use your fingers to spread out the first loop and push it flat against your head into a bow shape. Insert a bobby pin going from top to bottom and one going from bottom to top. Repeat on the other loop to finish the bow shape.

4. Pick part of the remaining end of the ponytail and wrap it up and around the hair elastic. This makes the middle of the bow.

5. Secure the middle of the bow with bobby pins underneath.

TIP

If your hair is thick, the sides of the bow can look a bit limp from the weight of the hair. Spray medium-hold hairspray on the loops before pinning it into place to coarsen the hair and help it stay upright.

70. FRENCH TWIST

BEST FOR

|||||| STRAIGHT

Nothing says "classic" like a beautiful French twist. The hair is pulled back away from the face and twisted into a gorgeous, elegant roll. The French twist works beautifully on chemically textured hair because you need a bit of texture to help hold the twist in place. I also love this look on straight hair so you can clearly see the roll. This style is perfect for mid-length hair. You can rock a French twist on a number of occasions but it is best suited to formal affairs. Don't feel left out if you don't have chemically textured hair; just spritz a little spray gel in your locks before blow drying and you will instantly get the texture you need to hold this style in place.

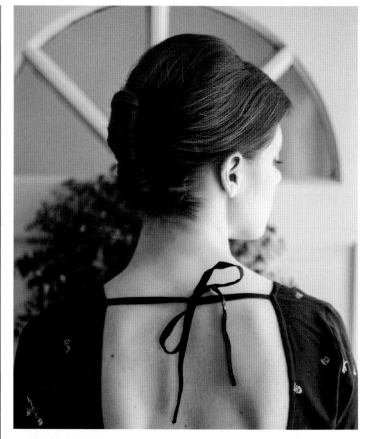

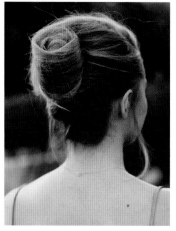

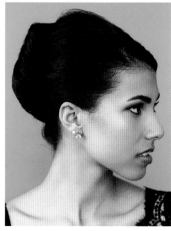

▶ **SEE ALSO**
Half-up bouffant,
page 102

HOW TO DO IT

WHAT YOU NEED

 PARTNER

- Comb
- Bobby pins
- Firm-hold hairspray

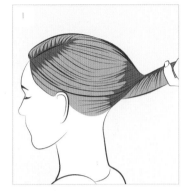

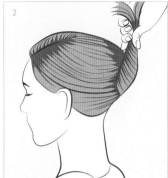

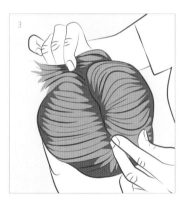

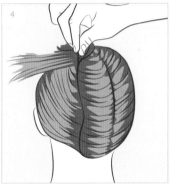

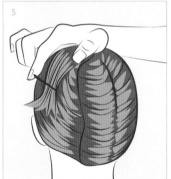

1. Pull all of your hair back toward the crown and hold it away from your head. Take the hair into your hands and tightly twist it in one direction.

2. Pull up your twist to create a roll shape on your head.

3. Start bobby pinning the roll to your head with the ends out.

4. To fix the roll neatly to the head, take the tip of the bobby pin downward, gripping onto the hair and then pushing it into your roll to make it tight.

5. At this point, you will probably have some hair sticking out of your roll. Take each section of hair, secure a bobby pin to the ends, and push it into the roll. Finish off this look with a firm-hold hairspray.

TIP

If you have a lot of flyaways and you're after a smoother texture, try using a shine spray. After styling, hold the shine spray 6-8 in (15-20 cm) away from your hair and spray over your rough ends.

71. VICTORY ROLLS

BEST FOR

 CURLY

 WAVY

It's true what they say—oldies are goodies, and this adorable vintage style from the 1940s is definitely a goodie. Victory rolls can be worn on a number of occasions including vintage-inspired parties, Halloween, and even holiday celebrations. It's an easy classic hairstyle that works best with mid-length to long hair because you need sufficient hair to form the rolls. For this look, you'll either need naturally wavy hair or to curl your hair first with a curling iron—then the roll will be lovely and defined.

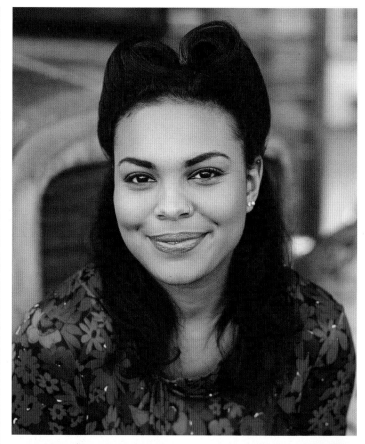

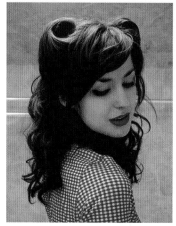

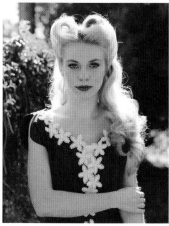

▶ **SEE ALSO**
Pompadour roll,
page 116

HOW TO DO IT

WHAT YOU NEED

- 1-in (2.5-cm) curling iron
- Bobby pins
- Firm-hold hairspray

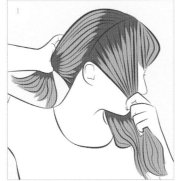

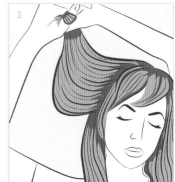

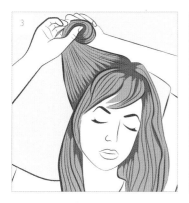

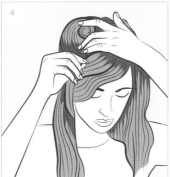

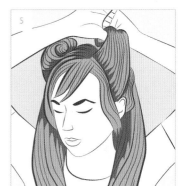

1. If your hair is naturally straight, add some curls with the curling iron, pointing it horizontally to create a nice wave (see glamour waves, page 112). Separate your hair from in front of the ears to use in your "roll." Brush out this section thoroughly.

2. Hold the section of hair out at a 45-degree angle and wrap it around your fingers to create the beginning of your roll.

3. Continue to roll the hair toward the scalp.

4. Once you have rolled the hair all the way up, pin it into place using bobby pins.

5. Repeat this same technique on the other side and pin into place. Spray your hair with a firm-hold hairspray so that it stays in place.

TIP

If your hair is really soft, try adding texture by applying a medium-hold hairspray and lightly teasing the hair, which will help you to roll it more easily.

72. BEEHIVE

BEST FOR

 CURLY

 FRIZZY

THICK

The modern beehive is a fun, flirty hairstyle that will work for several occasions, including dressy and formal. This do works best on thick, frizzy, or curly hair, which naturally provides the volume you need for a statement beehive. It also works beautifully with long hair—you will have the length needed to wrap around your ponytail, again creating the fullness you need for a true beehive. If you don't have naturally frizzy or curly hair, feel free to add some curls (see page 28) before getting started.

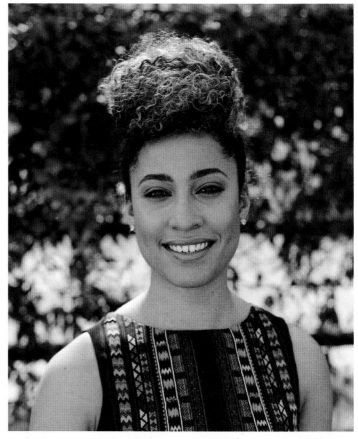

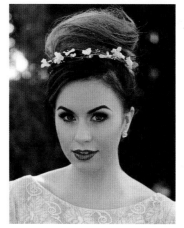

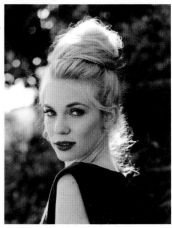

▶ **SEE ALSO**
Bouffant bun, page 94

HOW TO DO IT

WHAT YOU NEED

- Comb
- Hair elastics
- Medium-hold hairspray

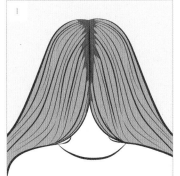

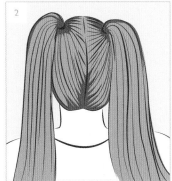

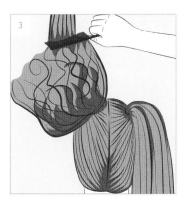

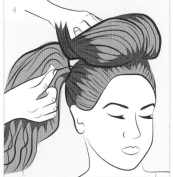

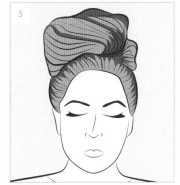

1. Start off with dry hair. Divide your hair in half from the center of your hairline back to the nape of the neck.

2. Create two ponytails right on the top of your crown, next to each other.

3. Starting with one pony, aggressively tease your hair from roots to ends with your comb. Repeat the same technique on the other ponytail.

4. Wrap one teased ponytail across the front of your hairline, securing it as you go with bobby pins.

5. Now wrap the second ponytail across the back of your hair, and secure it with bobby pins. Finish off the look by using a medium-hold hairspray.

TIP

You can dress up this look by adding a simple hair embellishment, brooch, or headband. This will make your modern beehive stand out even more!

73. GLAMOUR WAVES

BEST FOR

 STRAIGHT

 FINE

WAVY

CURLY

Glamour waves are a beautiful polished style that makes a great alternative to the typical beach waves look. This look is great for ladies with straight, fine hair—it will make their fine locks look bouncy and full. I also love this look on hair that has been colored and has some chemical texture, which will help the curl to stay and prevent it from falling flat. Curly-haired friends: don't feel left out. Simply round brush out your curls before creating this look.

▶ **SEE ALSO**
Beach waves, page 24

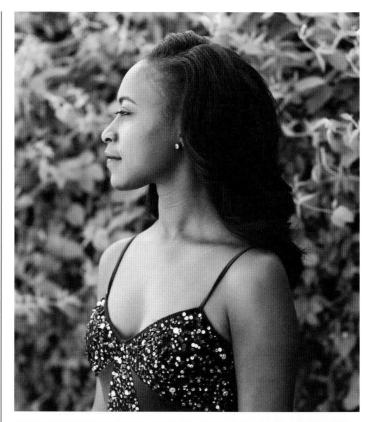

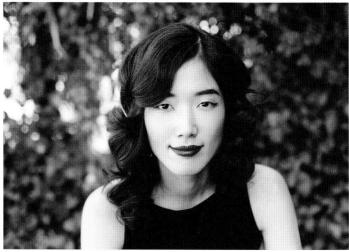

HOW TO DO IT

WHAT YOU NEED

 PARTNER

- Comb
- 1–2-in (2.5–5-cm) curling iron
- A few duck-bill clips
- Firm-hold hairspray

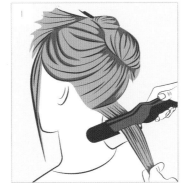

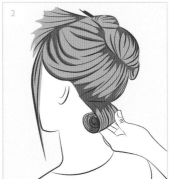

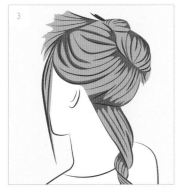

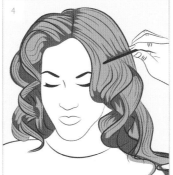

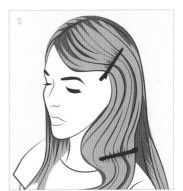

1. Make sure your hair is completely dry. Starting at the nape of the neck, section your hair directly below the ear from one side to the other. Hold the curling iron horizontally to the head, clamp down at the root area, and slowly ease the hair through the hair tong.

2. Allow the curl to cool down by holding the hair in place, or pin it up.

3. Once the curl is cool to touch, release it.

4. Continue using the same technique throughout the head, working up the nape of the neck to the top and sides of the hair. Once the hair is fully curled, lightly comb it out.

5. Where the curl bends, use a duck-bill clip to help set the wave. Continue to add the clips where the hair dips, creating an "S" formation. Keep the clips in the hair for a few minutes and then spray with a firm-hold hairspray to finish.

TIP

If your hair doesn't hold curl well, blow dry in a mousse for hold and texture then use a small curling iron to create small curls. The curls will soon drop and most likely produce the right amount of curl.

74. HIGH BOUFFANT PONY

BEST FOR

 FLAT

 FINE

This pony is no ordinary ponytail. It's a bit dressier than a standard ponytail and works best for ladies who have limp hair that naturally falls flat. Since you have to tease the root area in order to create a lot of height in this style, it will make the hair appear fuller. This look also works beautifully on hair that is mid-length to long with minimal short layers because after you create your bouffant, you tend to lose a little length in your ponytail. The high bouffant pony is just as suitable for a day in the office as for a night out on the town.

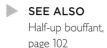 **SEE ALSO**
Half-up bouffant, page 102

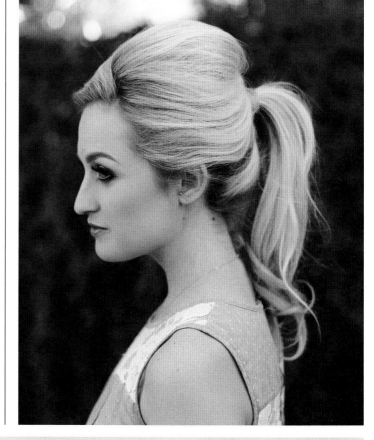

75. BARDOT POUF WITH LOW BUN

You can easily sweep up the back of your hair to create a gorgeous Bardot pouf with low bun to transform your hairstyle from day to evening in a matter of minutes. This look is great for ladies who have long hair and lack fullness because it gives your hair volume. Twist the hair from your ponytail and wrap it around the base of the pony to create a bun. Secure the bun into place with a few bobby pins. Finish off the look with medium-hold hairspray.

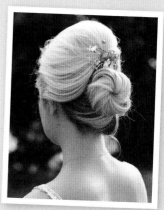

HOW TO DO IT

WHAT YOU NEED

- Comb
- Hair clip
- Hair elastics
- A few bobby pins
- Firm-hold hairspray

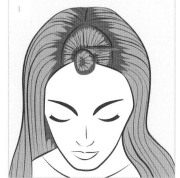

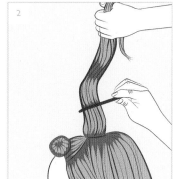

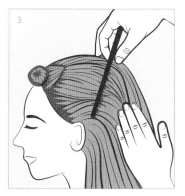

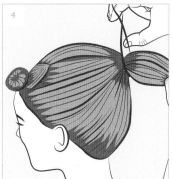

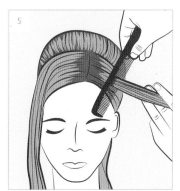

1. Create a small triangle section on top of the head from the crown to the sides of your hairline and clip it up to keep it out of the way.

2. Tease the top of your hair from a few inches away from the hairline to the crown of the head. If your hair is silky, use a little hairspray first.

3. Gently comb out the top of the backcombed hair toward the crown.

4. Twist the hair together near the low crown area, push it up, and lock into place with a bobby pin. If your hair is thick, use a few pins. Gather the remaining hair up to the twist and make a ponytail with an elastic.

5. Drop out the small triangle section, part it, and backcomb it slightly to give it volume. Then swoop it back toward the ponytail and pin in place. Take a small piece of hair from underneath the ponytail, wrap it around your ponytail, and secure the ends with a bobby pin. Use a firm-hold hairspray to finish off the look.

TIP

When backcombing the hair, tease from the mid-shaft of the hair down to the roots, which will give a lot of volume. If your hair is resistant to teasing, use a powder dust at the roots for extra hold and volume.

115

76. POMPADOUR ROLL

BEST FOR

 FINE

 FLAT

WAVY

FRIZZY

Calling all vintage enthusiasts: the pompadour hairstyle is for you! This style is unique and works beautifully paired with a vintage dress. You can also add some hair padding to the front to add height and hold the roll in place (see page 182). This look is ideal for anyone who has limp hair—the sock bun will instantly make your hair appear a lot fuller. It also looks lovely with frizzy hair; your natural frizziness emphasizes the roll at the front. This style works perfectly for mid-length to long hair with minimal layers around the face since you need enough length to wrap around the sock bun without layers falling out.

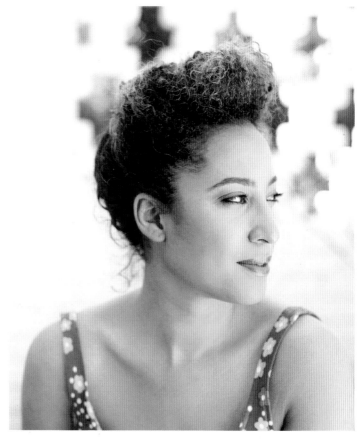

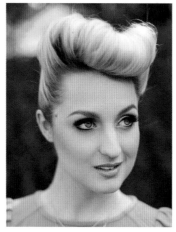

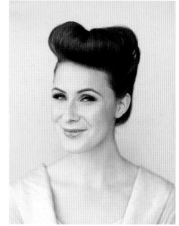

▶ **SEE ALSO**

Victory rolls, page 108

HOW TO DO IT

WHAT YOU NEED

- Sock-bun donut
- Scissors
- Hair clip
- Hair elastic
- Bobby pins
- Firm-hold hairspray

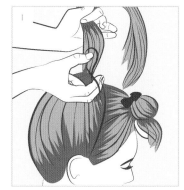
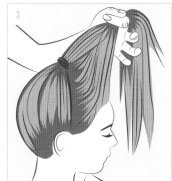
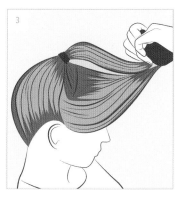
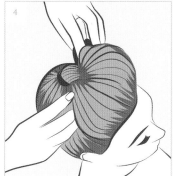
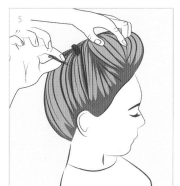

1. Cut the sock-bun donut on one side to create a long roll. Divide your hair from front to back and clip back the front section. Create a very high pony in front of your crown area by brushing all of your hair up toward the crown, gathering the hair, and securing it with a hair elastic.

2. Release the section of hair in front and add it to the hair at the back, combing it forward toward your face.

3. Take the cut sock bun, place it at the ends of the hair, and roll it toward the hairline.

4. Continue to roll the sock bun until it's tight to the head, creating a curved shape front of the face. This is the front of your pompadour.

5. Once the pompadour is in the place you want it, secure it with a few bobby pins. Finish off the look with a firm-hold hairspray.

TIP

When choosing your sock bun, note that there are several different colors so make sure to buy one that matches your hair color.

77. BUBBLE PONY

BEST FOR

  THICK

STRAIGHT

The bubble pony is a creative style, a little edgy, and packed with fun—perfect to wear for a rock concert or a night out with the girls. For this style, you make your hair appear fuller in desired areas, creating a bubble look. This look is suitable for long hair because when you tease the inside of the bubble, you will lose some length at the ends. It's most successful if your hair is thick, allowing you to achieve a very full bubble pony. I also recommend this look for straight hair so you can see the full bubble in the pony. If your hair isn't thick, you can use a hair thickening mousse prior to blow drying.

▶ **SEE ALSO**
Half-up bouffant,
page 102

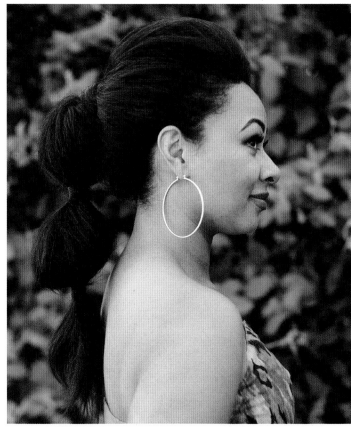

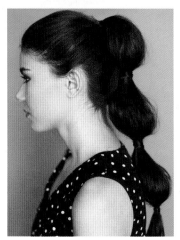

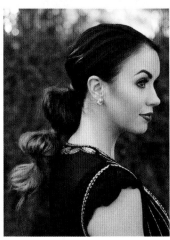

HOW TO DO IT

WHAT YOU NEED

 PARTNER

- Brush
- Hair elastics
- Hair clip
- Comb
- Hair powder (optional)
- Medium-hold hairspray

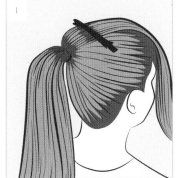

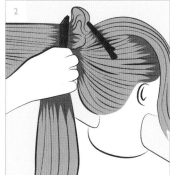

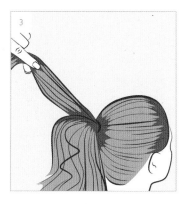

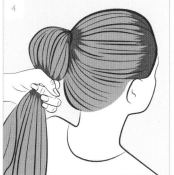

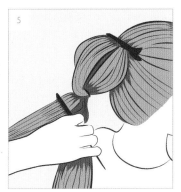

1. Brush your hair up and back into your crown area, make a ponytail, and secure it with a hair elastic. (If your hair is really thick, use two elastics.) Clip back a small section of hair from the top of your pony.

2. With the comb, aggressively tease the hair in your pony at the base of the hair elastic. If your hair is resistant to teasing, add hair powder.

3. Drop the clipped-back section over your teased section of hair and smooth it over. You may need to comb your hair over the teased section to smooth it.

4. Tie a hair elastic a few inches away from the first to make a bubble.

5. Create the second bubble by repeating the first steps: clip back a small section, tease the underneath hair and release the top section, smooth the hair over it and secure with a hair elastic. Repeat the bubble technique to make further bubbles and finish with hairspray.

TIP

If your hair isn't very long, feel free to add a few hair wefts at the base of your ponytail to create length.

78. GATSBY WAVES

BEST FOR

≡ FINE

||||| STRAIGHT

ξξξξ WAVY

The Gatsby waves style looks like it's difficult to achieve, but this version is so straightforward that you can transform yourself with this glamourous vintage style in minutes. The look works best if you have collarbone to mid-length hair because it will spring up and look shorter, true to the Gatsby look. It is most successful if your hair is on the fine side. When you curl it, you'll create a lot of fullness. You could rock this look at a vintage-themed party or any holiday function.

▷ SEE ALSO
Glamour waves,
page 112

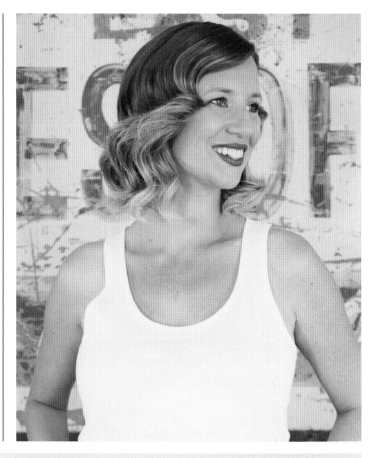

79. FAUX BOB

This style hides a secret—this girl actually has long, fine hair. It's perfect if you want to keep your long locks but occasionally wear a short style. You can create a faux bob by curling your hair as for the Gatsby waves, then adding a loose braid from the shoulders downward, and tucking the braid underneath the hair. Secure your braid with bobby pins to keep the faux bob in place.

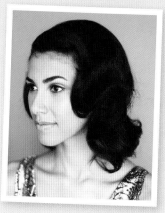

HOW TO DO IT

WHAT YOU NEED

 PARTNER

- Hair clip
- 1-in (2.5-cm) curling iron
- Duck-bill clips
- Firm-hold hairspray

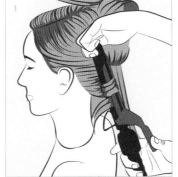

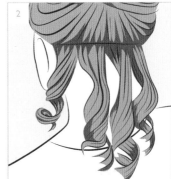

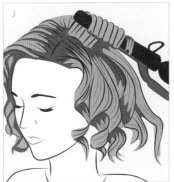

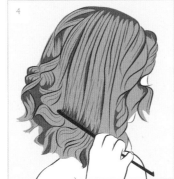

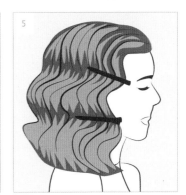

1. Section your hair from ear to ear. In the bottom section, curl 1–2-in (2.5–5-cm) sections of your hair with the curling iron. Hold your iron vertical, clamping at the hair root and easing the hair through the hair tong. Allow it to sit for 2–3 seconds and release.

2. Curl the rest of the bottom section in small sections.

3. Continue this technique all throughout the head, sectioning your hair and curling your hair in 1–2-in (2.5–5-cm) sections, making sure you always curl in the same direction.

4. Lightly comb out your hair.

5. Comb downward into the crease of the curl, then add a duck-bill clip in the crease. This will help your wave form. Clip the next crease too, and then clip the rest of your hair in the same way. Hairspray your hair and let it sit for a few minutes to take the shape. Release the clips.

TIP

For this style, check that you are always pointing your iron vertically—if you point it horizontally, you will create glamour waves (see page 112).

CHAPTER 5
EXTRA SPECIAL

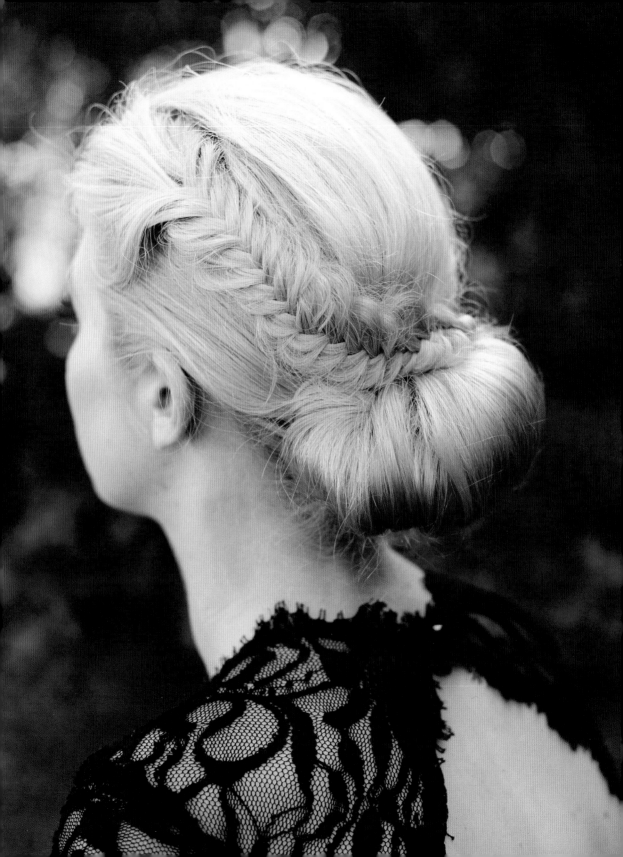

80. LOW TWISTED UPDO

BEST FOR

 WAVY

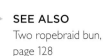 CURLY

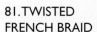 THICK

This twisted updo is great for
beginners because you simply
twist the hair and pin it into place.
It works beautifully for women
who have thick hair because the
twists make the hair appear less
bulky. I also love this look on
wavy hair because when you
twist the hair, the natural curl will
give your twists definition. This
style is best for mid-length
hair— the twist will be the
perfect size. Fine-haired girls can
rock this look as well—just add
some dry shampoo before you
start so your hair looks thicker.

▶ **SEE ALSO**
Two ropebraid bun,
page 128

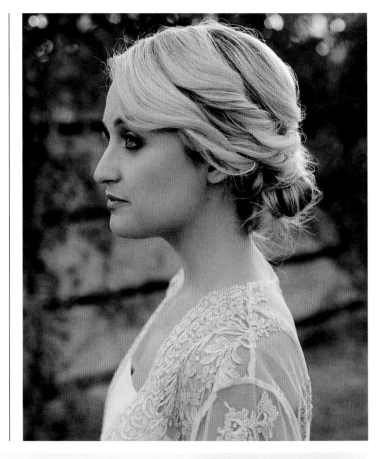

81. TWISTED FRENCH BRAID

If you've fallen in love with the
low twisted updo, you'll love
this style, which combines a
twisted updo with a French
braid. This look is great for
thick hair because the twist
helps condense the thickness.
Take three small sections and
twist them. Take the right one
up and over into the middle,
then the left one up and over
to the middle. Incorporate
small sections of hair using the
French braid technique (see
page 80), working from right
to left down the back of the
head, and twisting each
section before adding it to
the braid. Secure the ends
with a hair elastic.

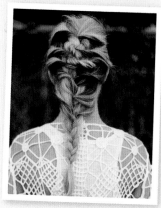

HOW TO DO IT

WHAT YOU NEED

- Comb
- Clips
- Bobby pins
- Firm-hold hairspray
- Spray shine (optional)

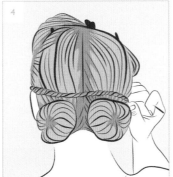
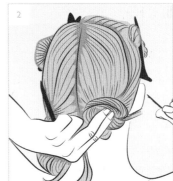
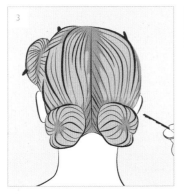
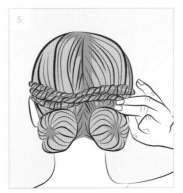
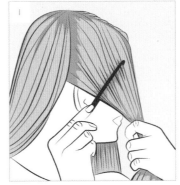

1. Start with dry hair that hasn't been washed for a day or two. Clip back the front sections in front of the ears.

2. Working with the back of the hair first, make two twisted buns. To do this, split the hair in half, clip back the left section, and twist the right section as much as you can until it starts to coil, creating a bun effect. Secure it with bobby pins.

3. Drop out your left section and repeat.

4. Release the front sections and divide them into two or three smaller sections. Take the first 1–2-in (2.5–5-cm) section. Working from the bottom, twist it away from the face toward the back of your hair, take it to the opposite side, and secure it in place with a bobby pin.

5. Repeat with the other sections until you have no more hair to work with. Finish with firm-hold hairspray, or shine spray for smoothness.

TIP

If your hair is very thick, you can make three to five buns in Step 2.

125

82. KNOTTED FAUX HAWK

BEST FOR

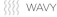 THICK

WAVY

FLAT

While most braids and knots are soft and simple, sometimes we want our edgy side to shine. The knotted faux hawk gives a hint of elegance with a whole lot of spice. Yet achieving this sassy style involves nothing more complicated than making a basic knot. The knotted faux hawk style works best on thick hair that is chemically textured. It is also great for flat hair because the knots add bulk to your hair. I recommend this look if you have mid-length hair, which will produce several knots but not too many. If your hair isn't wavy or chemically textured, use a spray gel or mousse before drying your hair, and add some waves (see beach waves tutorial, page 24).

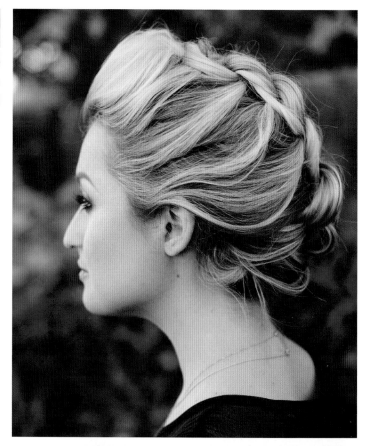

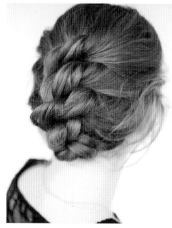

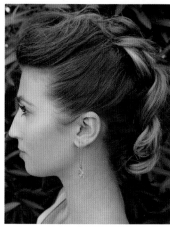

▶ **SEE ALSO**
Dutch braid faux hawk, page 138

HOW TO DO IT

WHAT YOU NEED

- Comb
- Hair elastic
- Bobby pins

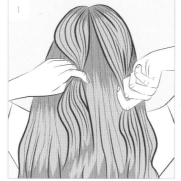

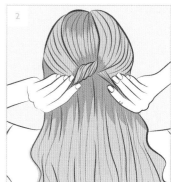

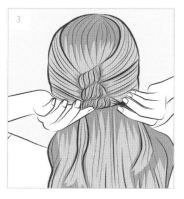

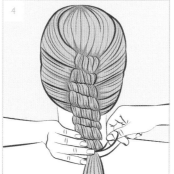

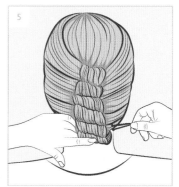

1. Make sure your hair is free of tangles and knots. Grab a section of hair on each side of your head, a few inches away from your hairline.

2. Take the two sections of hair and make a simple knot.

3. Take another section of hair from each side of the head, incorporate them into the previous sections, and create another knot.

4. Work this same technique down to the nape of the neck. When you run out of hair to connect, continue knotting your hair until you reach the ends and secure with a hair elastic.

5. Roll the end of the hair up under itself, tuck it under the knots, and pin to secure. If you want a fuller effect, simply tug on each knot to give a tad more bulk to the texture.

TIP

If you are left with an extremely long knotted pony, and you're struggling to tuck the end in under your faux hawk, you can always let it fall straight down.

83. TWO ROPEBRAID BUN

BEST FOR

 THICK

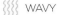 WAVY

 CURLY

 FRIZZY

The two ropebraid bun brings plenty of fullness to the average bun. You can wear this upstyle for any business occasion. The two ropebraid bun is perfect for ladies who have extremely thick hair that is wavy or curly. The ropebraids condense the bulk of the hair and because the hair is braided before you make the bun, it helps your hair stay in place. This style works beautifully for frizzy hair too; little wispy bits can add to the look. You'll need long hair for this style—at least 8 in (20 cm) of hair is required to create a dramatic ropebraid. This hairstyle is just right for a formal occasion.

▶ **SEE ALSO**
Ropebraid bun,
page 54

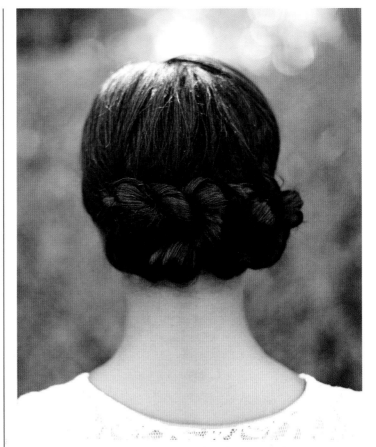

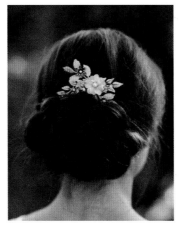

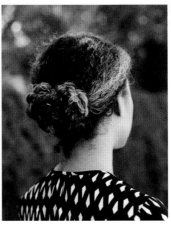

HOW TO DO IT

WHAT YOU NEED

- Brush
- 4 hair elastics
- Bobby pins
- Medium-hold hairspray

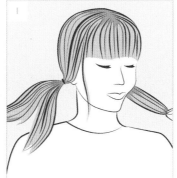
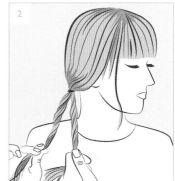
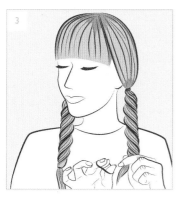
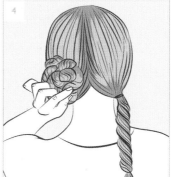
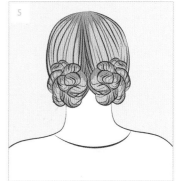

1. Start with dry hair. Split the hair in half down the center. Create two pigtails (see page 70).

2. Inside each pigtail, split the hair in half and create a ropebraid (see page 20).

3. Continue until you get to the ends and secure with a hair elastic.

4. Wrap the first ropebraid around the hair elastic to create a bun and secure it with a few bobby pins.

5. Make the other ropebraid bun right next to the first. Finish off the look with a medium-hold hairspray.

TIP

If you want your ropebraid buns to be full and messy, spray a lightweight hairspray onto your hair before you start, and massage the hair out a little. This will help create lots of little wispy bits.

84. CRISS-CROSS FRENCH BRAID UPDO

BEST FOR

 THICK

STRAIGHT

 WAVY

We usually think of braids draping across our back. People rarely think of braided updos. If you know how to do a French braid, you can easily achieve a flirty French-braided updo. Pinning up the braids makes an elegant hairstyle that works well for ladies with thick hair; braiding the hair tightly to the head reduces much of the bulk. It's also great for mid-length hair so that the braids criss-cross neatly at the neck. This braided do works beautifully with straight to wavy hair so you can see the definition in the braid.

▶ **SEE ALSO**
French braid, page 80

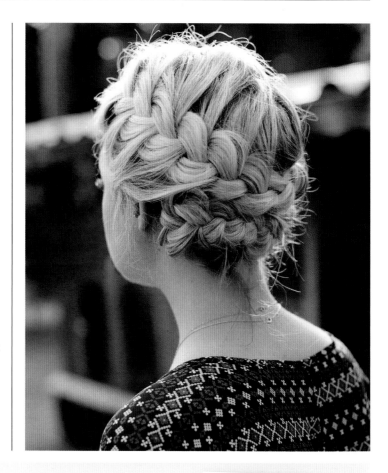

85. FRENCH BRAID UPDO

You can easily get a different look to the criss-cross French braid updo. This look suits fine hair that has a slight wave to it. Instead of doing two French braids, you do one French braid, starting from the front of the hairline and going toward the nape of the neck. Then tuck the end of the braid under your hair at the neck, securing it with bobby pins. Use medium-hold hairspray to finish.

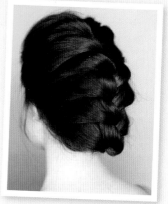

HOW TO DO IT

WHAT YOU NEED

- Brush
- 2 hair elastics
- A few bobby pins
- Firm-hold hairspray

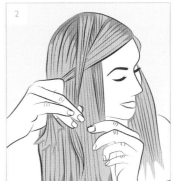

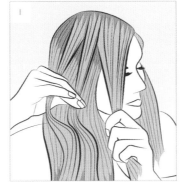

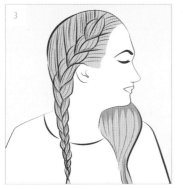

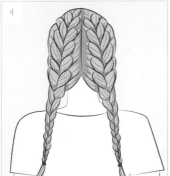

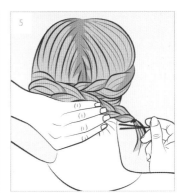

1. Make sure your hair is free of tangles before starting. Part your hair on the desired side from front to back. Starting on the right side of your head, split the front part of your hair into three sections.

2. Follow the French braid technique (see page 80), following your hairline down the side of your face.

3. Once you reach the nape of the neck, continue with a three-strand braiding technique (see page 51). When you reach the ends, secure with a hair elastic.

4. Repeat on the other side, working the sections left to right.

5. Take the hanging ends that are left, cross them over each other, and secure them with bobby pins. Use firm-hold hairspray to finish.

TIP

Feel free to get creative and try the Dutch braid (see page 90) for this hairstyle. You can pull out the braid slightly to add volume.

86. DUTCH BRAID WITH ROPEBRAID UPDO

BEST FOR

 THICK

STRAIGHT

WAVY

FRIZZY

The Dutch braid with ropebraid updo consists of two techniques in one—a soft, romantic ropebraid bun at the back, overlapped by two pancaked Dutch braids. You can wear this style for a variety of occasions but I prefer wearing it with a sophisticated dress. You need to have long hair for this one so you have enough length for your ropebraids to wrap across the back of the bun. I also love it on thick hair, which creates large, dramatic braids. It's perfect for frizzier hair too; the Dutch braids and ropebraid help tame your hair and keep it neatly in position. If you hair is fine, you can add a thickening mousse before you start and once you've made the braids, pull them out at the sides a little so they appear thicker.

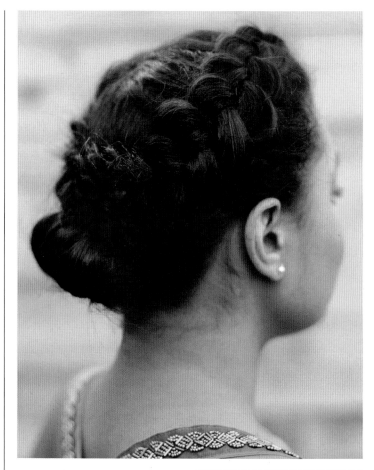

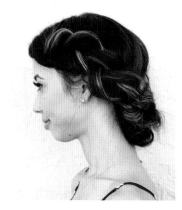

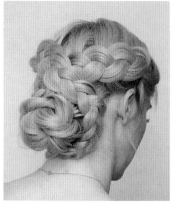

▶ **SEE ALSO**
Dutch braid, page 90

HOW TO DO IT

WHAT YOU NEED

 PARTNER

- Comb
- Hair elastics
- Bobby pins
- Hair clips
- Spray wax or dry shampoo (optional)

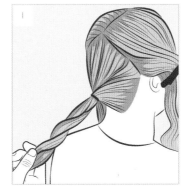

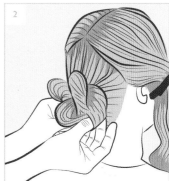

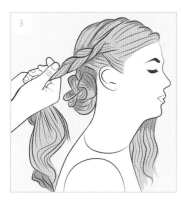

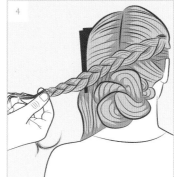

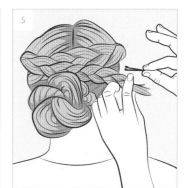

1. Take a section from the low crown to the tip of your ear on each side to create triangle sections and clip them back. Make a low pony at the nape of the neck. Divide it into two sections and create a ropebraid by taking the section to the right, twisting it to the right, and taking it over to the left side. Repeat until you reach about 1 in (2.5 cm) from the ends (see page 20). Secure with a hair elastic.

2. Twist the ropebraid up around the hair elastic. Bobby pin in place.

3. Drop out the top sections and part on one side. Split the hair in half and make a Dutch braid (see page 90).

4. When you reach halfway across your head, do a three-strand braid (see page 51) to the end. Repeat on the other side. Secure the ends with a hair elastic.

5. Wrap the braided sections across one another and pin into place.

TIP

If your hair is clean or very fine, use spray wax or dry shampoo to create bulk. It will also prevent your braid from going limp. Also, gently tug on each strand of the braid to make it look fuller.

87. RODARTE BRAID

BEST FOR

 FINE

WAVY

All braid enthusiasts love a good Rodarte braid. This style became popular after it graced the runway and has been going strong ever since. This look is on the bohemian side and is great for outdoor concerts or other al fresco events. The Rodarte braid is best on long hair with few layers because you need the length to create a dramatic rose and a long braid. It also works well for fine hair with some waves in it, whether natural or created with the curling iron. If you like, you can pull out the braid a little at the sides for a thicker appearance.

▶ **SEE ALSO**
Flower bun, page 100

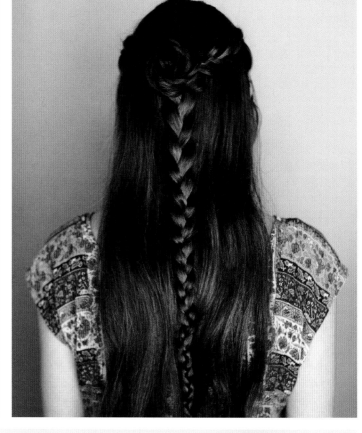

88. RODARTE INTO ONE BRAID

Change up your look by turning your Rodarte braid into a fun side-braided style. To create a dramatic side braid, you'll need to have long hair. Follow the steps opposite to create a Rodarte braid. Then gather all of your hair to one side and simply braid your hair into a three-strand braid (see page 51). Secure the ends with a hair elastic and finish off the look by using a medium-hold hairspray.

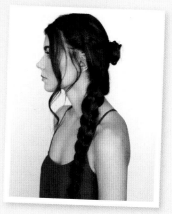

HOW TO DO IT

WHAT YOU NEED

 PARTNER

- Comb
- 4 hair elastics
- Hair clip
- Flexible-hold hairspray

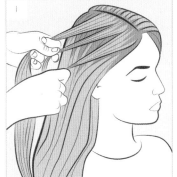

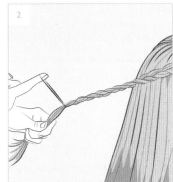

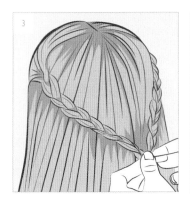

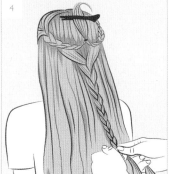

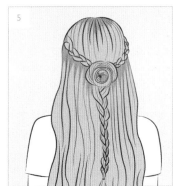

1. Part your hair on the desired side and divide a small section of hair into three equal sections.

2. Create a simple three-strand braid (see page 51). Continue until you have 3–4 in (7.5–10 cm) of hair left and secure the ends with a hair elastic. Make a similar braid on the other side.

3. Pull both braids to the crown of the head and secure them with a hair elastic.

4. Clip the braid upward and create another simple braid directly underneath the two connected braids. Secure the ends with a hair elastic.

5. Release the clip. Using the hair left out of the hair elastic, make a three-strand braid and then create a rose shape by winding it into a circle. Bobby pin the rose into place at the base of your braid. Use hairspray to finish.

TIP

This hairstyle is great for second-day hair. Spray a bit of dry shampoo into it before getting started and you're good to go.

89. TWISTED WATERFALL BRAID

BEST FOR

 THICK

 WAVY

 CURLY

FRIZZY

This style is literally a standard waterfall braid with a twist. This look is fun, flirty, and bohemian. The twisted waterfall braid is suitable for mid-length to long hair and works best if your hair is quite thick, allowing you to show off the contrasting delicate waterfall braid. If your hair is on the finer side, the braid won't stand out as much. I also recommend this do for wavy, curly, or frizzy hair, which will help give it an ultra-boho vibe.

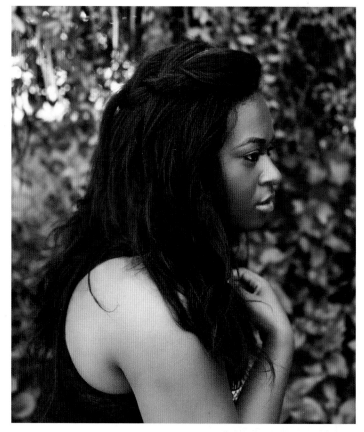

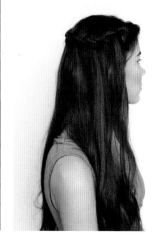

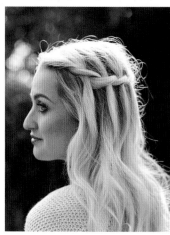

▶ **SEE ALSO**
Lace braid with waves, page 54

HOW TO DO IT

WHAT YOU NEED

 PARTNER

- Comb
- Hair elastic
- Bobby pin

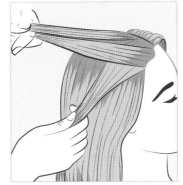

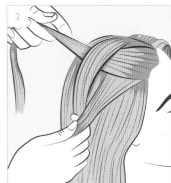

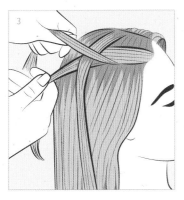

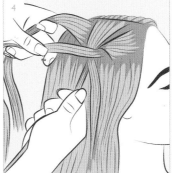

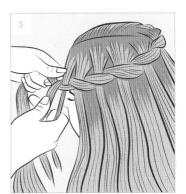

1. Take three sections of hair at the front hairline. Cross the lower section over the middle section, away from the face.

2. Take the section from the top of your head and let it down over the middle section, creating the "drop-out" section.

3. Twist the bottom section over the drop-out section, locking it into place and creating a ropebraid waterfall.

4. Lay another waterfall section from the top of your head over the top section of the ropebraid and twist the lower section over again.

5. Repeat this process until the braid is as long as you want. You can continue the braid to the other side of the head. If you still have hair left at the end, continue with a three-strand braid (see page 51) and secure with a hair elastic. To hide the end of the braid, tuck it underneath the braid and pin it into place with a bobby pin.

TIP

If your hair is silky before you start, your waterfall braid may fall out during the day. To avoid this, add a dry shampoo to create some grip and ensure your braid stays in place.

90. DUTCH BRAID FAUX HAWK

BEST FOR

 FINE

 STRAIGHT

$\{\{\{\}$ WAVY

This style is for the inner rocker in you—take a simple Dutch braid and make it into a rocker faux hawk. It's the perfect style for a night out or a rock concert. This style works well if you have some chemical texture, which will give your faux hawk the volume needed for this look. I prefer this look on ladies with straight or wavy hair so that you can clearly see the inside-out part of the braid. The Dutch braid faux hawk is also good for fine hair; you pull out the braid to make it appear thicker.

▶ **SEE ALSO**
Dutch braid, page 90

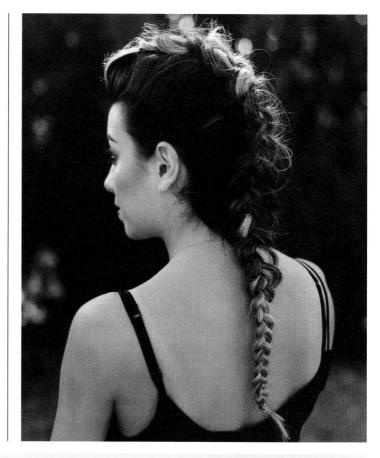

91. DUTCH BRAID UPDO

If a faux hawk isn't your thing, try to soften this look by using similar techniques but turn it into an elegant Dutch braid updo. This look works with fine hair—when you tuck up the ends you won't have too much bulk underneath. To soften the look, don't pancake your Dutch braid out as much as you would when doing the faux hawk. Then take the tail of your braid, tuck it in and under your Dutch braid and bobby pin it into place. Finish off the look with a medium-hold hairspray.

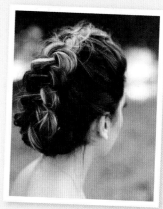

HOW TO DO IT

WHAT YOU NEED

 PARTNER

- Comb
- Hair elastic
- Firm-hold hairspray
- Shine spray (optional)

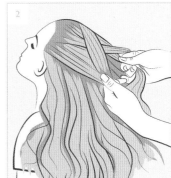

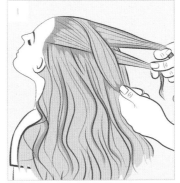

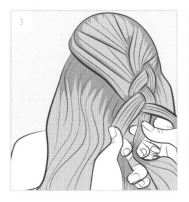

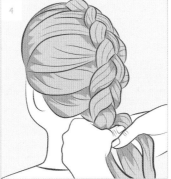

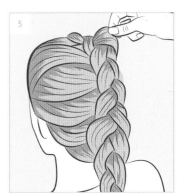

1. Tip your head back and divide the hair in three equal sections, 1–2 in (2.5–5 cm) away from the hairline. You work the Dutch-braid technique underhanded, so hold your fingers upward. Take the left section underneath into the middle. This is your new middle section.

2. Take the right side section and go underneath the middle section. This is your new middle section.

3. Add hair as you work toward the nape. First add a small section of hair on the left side into your left section and take that whole section into the middle. Repeat on the other side and keep alternating.

4. When you don't have any more hair to add, continue doing a normal three-strand braid (see page 51). Secure the ends with a hair elastic.

5. Pull on each side of your braid to create bulk and fullness. Finish this look by pulling your hair upward at the hairline and hairspraying it.

TIP

Sometimes when you pull the braid out you can create unwanted frizziness. If this happens, use shine spray to help smooth it down. Spray it all over the hair from 6-8 in (15-20 cm) away.

92. THREE-BRAIDED PRETZEL UPDO

BEST FOR

 THICK

 STRAIGHT

 WAVY

The three-braided pretzel bun braid is really easy but it looks really intricate. It's the perfect hairstyle for enthusiasts who have really thick hair and a hard time with updos. When you create three braids and tie them into one updo, you reduce the bulkiness of the hair. This hairstyle is also great for mid-length hair, which makes good-sized pretzels. It's also ideal for straight to wavy hair so you will see the definition in the braid. This style can be worn casually or dressed up for a fun night out.

▶ **SEE ALSO**
Two ropebraid
bun, page 128

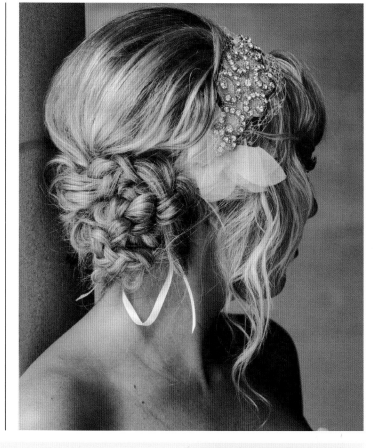

93. MESSY LOW BRAIDED BUN

You can easily achieve a totally different look with the messy low braided bun. This style is great for long, wavy hair—the waves naturally create a messy look. Simply create one large three-strand braid at the back and secure the ends with a hair elastic.

Gently pull at your braid to create a messy look, then wrap your braid into a bun, securing it into place using bobby pins. To create a few wisps around your face, gently massage your hair out of the bun with the palms of your hands.

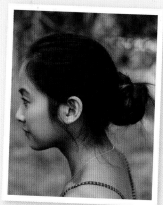

HOW TO DO IT

WHAT YOU NEED

 PARTNER

- Comb
- Hair elastics
- Bobby pins
- Medium-hold hairspray

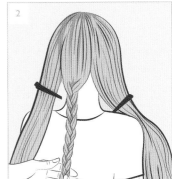

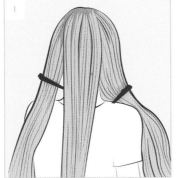

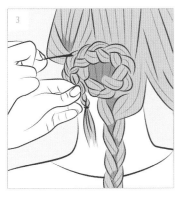

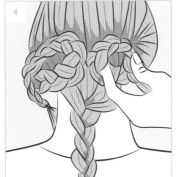

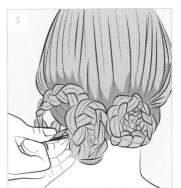

1. Divide your hair into three sections, one on each side and a section at the back.

2. Inside each section, braid the hair using a three-strand braiding technique (see page 51) and secure each braid with a hair elastic at the ends.

3. Starting on the left side, create a loop with the left-side section and take it to about halfway across your head. Secure the braid with bobby pins.

4. Take the right-side section and create a loop in the same way, crossing over from the right to the left, to about halfway across your head. Secure the braid with bobby pins.

5. Make a loop with the middle braid in between the first two loops and secure it with bobby pins. Finish off with hairspray.

TIP

If your hair is fine and you want to try this look, apply a dry shampoo for some extra fullness and stretch out your braid before pinning it up to make your hair look thicker.

94. HALF-CROWN DUTCH BRAID

BEST FOR

 WAVY

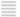 CURLY

FLAT

This is a very romantic-looking style that you can wear in various ways—casually or embellished with a floral piece for a smart occasion. It works beautifully if you have long hair with minimal layers. Your hair needs to be long enough for the braid to reach across your head without stray hairs coming out. It's a useful style to have in your repertoire if you have flat hair because the Dutch braids add volume around your head. I also love the look of this style on wavy or curly hair, which gives a bohemian touch.

 SEE ALSO
Brocade braid half style, page 32

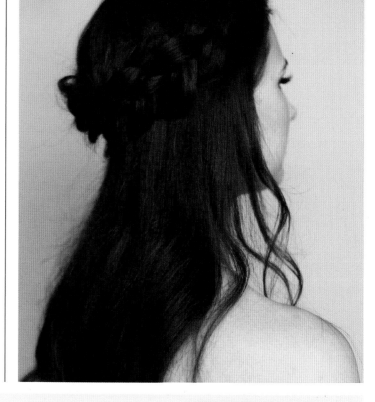

95. CROWN BRAID HALF STYLE

You can get a totally different look by not pinning the braid to the back of the head. For this look you will need long hair so you have enough hair to wrap across the forehead. Instead of making a Dutch braid, make a three-strand braid (see page 51) and wrap it across the forehead instead of at the back of the head. Secure the braid in place with bobby pins or a pretty clip.

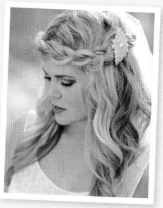

HOW TO DO IT

WHAT YOU NEED

 PARTNER

- Curling iron (optional)
- Comb
- 2 hair elastics
- Medium-hold hairspray

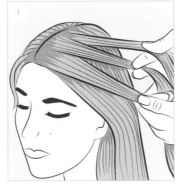

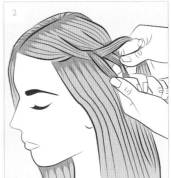

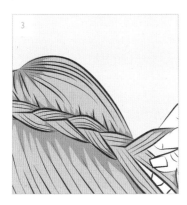

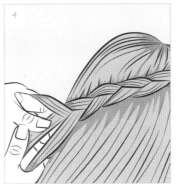

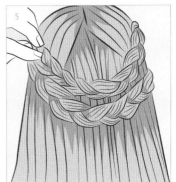

1. Start with dry hair. You can wear this style with straight hair or add some waves or curls to make the braid a little fuller (see pages 24 and 28). Part your hair on the desired side, take a 2-in (5-cm) section of hair at the parting and divide it into three.

2. Create a Dutch braid on the left side of your hair, working your braid underhanded (see page 90).

3. Incorporating hair from the right side of the braid only, braid until you get to the back of your head. If you have leftover hair, make a three-strand braid (see page 51). Secure the ends with a hair elastic.

4. Make a Dutch braid in the same way on the right side of your head. This time you will incorporate hair from the left side of the braid.

5. Take the ends of each braid, wrap them across the back of your head, and bobby pin into place. Finish with medium-hold hairspray.

TIP

If you have flyaways, use a shine spray to help soften and tame the frizziness. Hold 6-8 in (15-20 cm) away from the hair and spray generously.

96. INFINITY BUN

BEST FOR

 WAVY

FLAT

The infinity bun is a little bit daring and different. While this style is elegant, it's also unusual and works for alternative looks. It's easiest to achieve the infinity shape if your hair is wavy or chemically textured, it will help the bun to stay in place. It can work wonders for flat hair, providing dramatic interest at the back. If you don't have waves or chemical texture, add a mousse before blow drying for texture and create some waves with a curling iron.

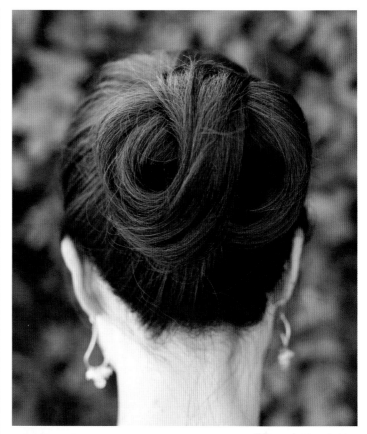

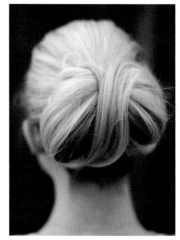

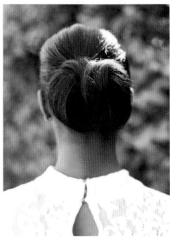

▶ **SEE ALSO**
Celtic knot, page 150

HOW TO DO IT

WHAT YOU NEED

 PARTNER

- Brush
- Hair elastic
- 5–10 bobby pins
- Firm-hold hairspray

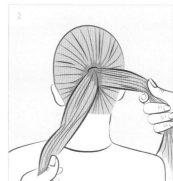

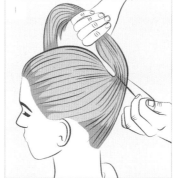

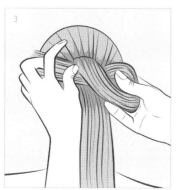

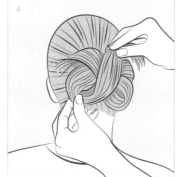

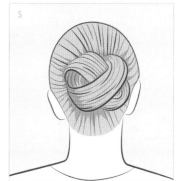

1. Brush your hair well, then brush it up and away from your face toward the low crown area. Gather all of your hair together and create a ponytail by securing it at the low crown area with a hair elastic.

2. Split the hair in half inside your ponytail, then twist the right-hand section to the right.

3. Create a large loop and wrap the ends around the other side. This will be half of your infinity sign. Bobby pin it into place.

4. Repeat on the other side by twisting the hair slightly to the left, creating a loop, wrapping the ends around the other side, and securing with bobby pins.

5. Use a firm-hold hairspray to ensure your style stays in place.

TIP

If your hair has layers, apply a pomade to the loops before you create the infinity shape to hold them in place and add some texture.

97. FIVE-STRAND BRAID

BEST FOR

|||||| STRAIGHT

〳〳〳 WAVY

Nothing says "statement braid" like the gorgeous five-strand braid. You can wear it several ways—off to the side, straight down the back, or even half up with some waves. The instructions may seem intimidating at first, but once you get the hang of the weaving pattern, you can easily create this braid. For this look, you'll need very long hair with minimal layers. You need lots of length to make a substantial five-strand braid, and if you have layers, they'll pop out of the braid. This look works best if your hair is straight or wavy so that the strands stand out. This look is versatile: wear it casually for a stroll on the beach or jazz it up with a hair embellishment to wear for a formal occasion.

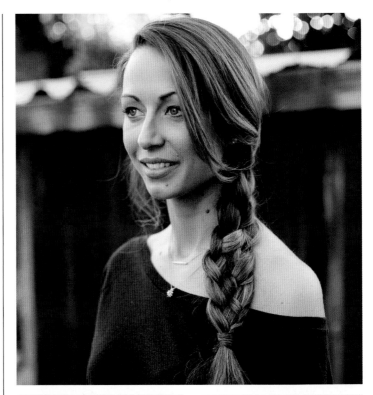

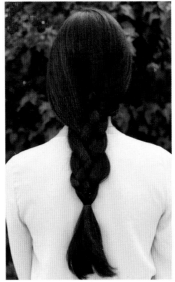

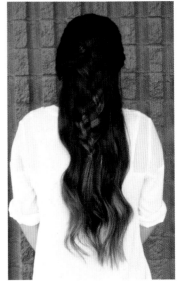

▷ **SEE ALSO**
Messy side braid, page 50

HOW TO DO IT

WHAT YOU NEED

  PARTNER

- Brush
- Hair elastic
- Hairspray (optional)

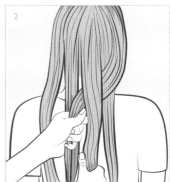

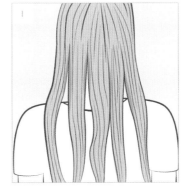

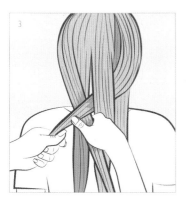

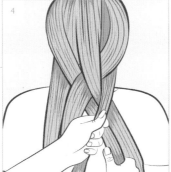

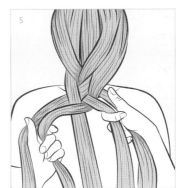

1. Start with dry hair, clean or dirty. Brush out the hair and get rid of any tangles or knots. Separate it into five even sections.

2. Take the outermost strand on the right and cross it over the strand to the left and under the middle strand. Leave the strand there. This is the new middle strand.

3. Take the outermost strand on the left, cross it over the strand to the right, and under the middle strand.

4. Repeat Step 2 on the right side again.

5. Repeat until the whole length of hair is braided, then secure with a hair elastic. Spritz with hairspray if desired.

TIP

If you find it difficult to start using the right strand, you can start with the left strand and reverse the instructions.

98. LOW ROLLED UPDO

BEST FOR

▨ STRAIGHT

▨ FINE

Nothing says "classy" like a gorgeous rolled updo. I love this hairstyle because you can finish it off in a number of ways. Feeling creative? Throw in some curls around the face or a simple braid to make a statement. If you have fine hair and want to make your hair look thicker, this is the style for you as when you tease your hair to make the roll, it creates volume. This style also works for straight hair, which gives you a tidy roll. If your hair isn't fine and you want to try this style, only tease your hair a little so you don't end up with a huge roll.

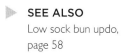 **SEE ALSO**
Low sock bun updo,
page 58

99. ROLLED UPDO WITH FISHTAIL BRAID

Pairing the rolled updo with a fishtail braid takes the elegance of the style up a notch. This works well with fine, mid-length hair. Before sectioning out your hair for the roll, take a large section from the side and clip it for later. Create your rolled updo, then make a fishtail braid (see page 38). Now wrap your completed braid over the rolled updo and secure the ends with a hair elastic.

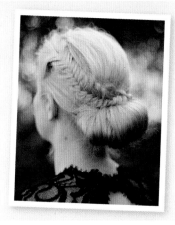

HOW TO DO IT

WHAT YOU NEED

 PARTNER

- Comb
- Hair clips
- Hair elastics
- Hairspray
- Bobby pins
- Firm-hold hairspray

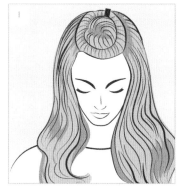

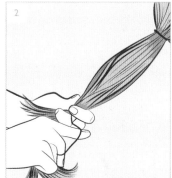

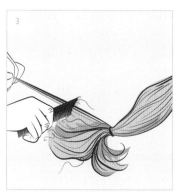

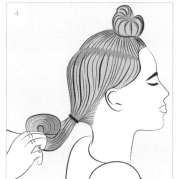

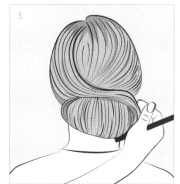

1. Start with smooth, dry hair. Section out a large triangle of hair from the crown of your head for later and clip it up.

2. Comb the rest of your hair back to the nape of your neck and create a low ponytail. Secure the top of the ponytail with one hair elastic and then add another 2–3 in (5–7.5 cm) from the bottom of your hair.

3. Backcomb the hair under the second elastic.

4. Starting at the bottom of your hair, roll in the ends tightly. Roll up the ponytail until you reach your head and pin with bobby pins to create your updo.

5. Unclip the section of hair at the front of your head and part on the desired side. Wrap one side of your hair back round your head and over the top of the updo, neatly tucking the ends away and securing with bobby pins. Repeat on the other side. Finish off with hairspray.

TIP

To make your rolled updo appear smoother, apply pomade on your palms, rub them together, and run them over the areas where you have flyaways. This will give some added shine and leave your hair frizz free.

100. CELTIC KNOT

BEST FOR

THICK
STRAIGHT
WAVY

The Celtic knot is the perfect hairstyle for my minimalist friends. You can wear your hair down and make a huge statement by adding a Celtic knot at the back. It's a simple, natural look for a wedding or other festive affair, or you could wear it casually with a bohemian outfit. This hairstyle looks best with thick hair because the Celtic knot will be large and show up well. You also need to have long hair with minimal layers. You can still wear a Celtic knot if you have fine hair, but it won't be as defined.

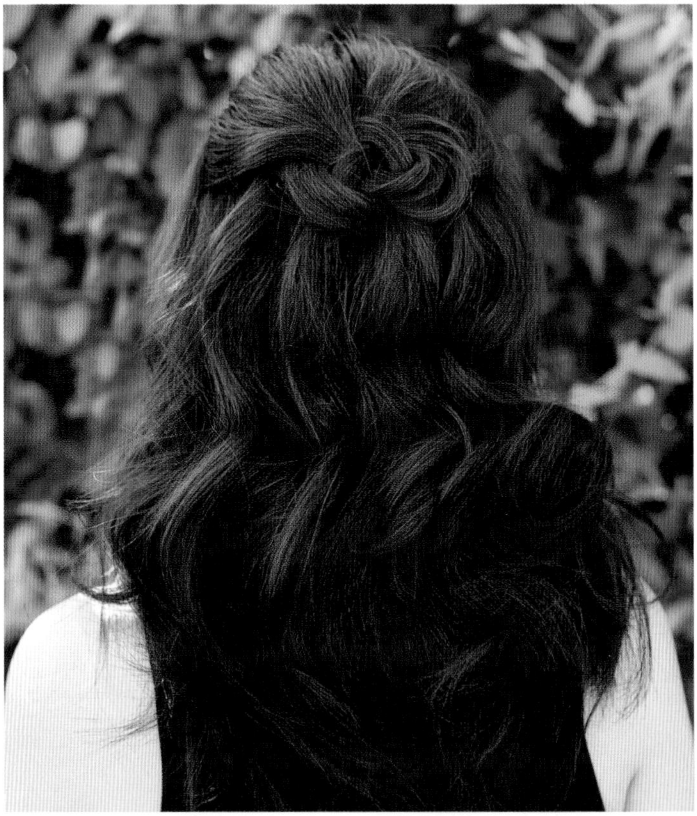

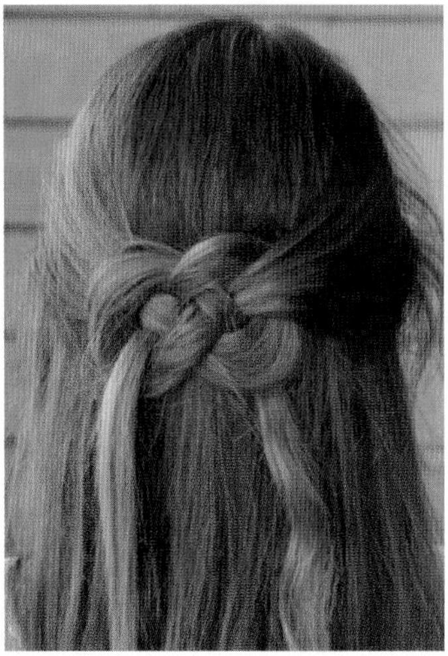

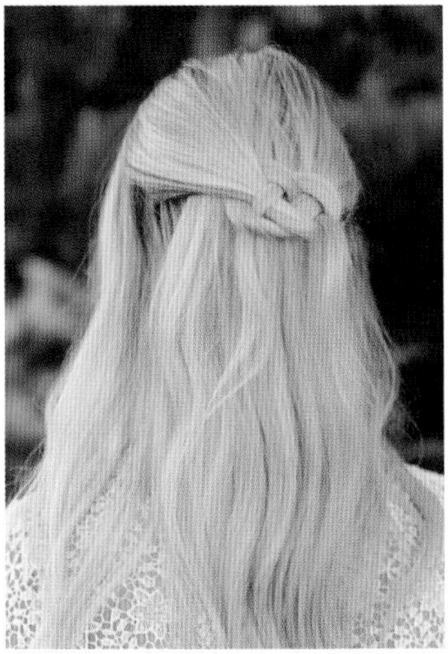

SEE ALSO
Flower bun, page 100

HOW TO DO IT

WHAT YOU NEED

 PARTNER

- Brush
- Hairspray (optional)

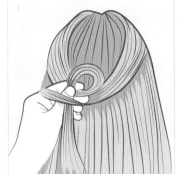

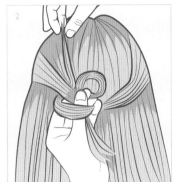

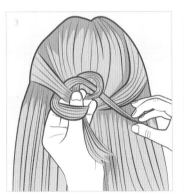

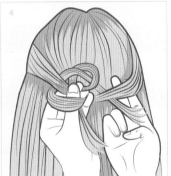

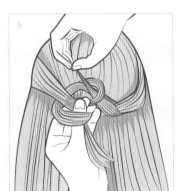

1. Brush out any tangles. Take a large section of hair from the left part of your head to make a loop on one side of your hair. Take a section from the other side and put it under the loop.

2. Pull this section of hair under the other one, keeping it tight.

3. Roll this section of hair under the first one, pulling it through the loop as shown.

4. Tuck the end of the hair under the section of hair on the right.

5. Bring the hair back up and over the right-hand section of hair and pull the hair through the loop. Find the bottom of the loop and pull the two ends to fix the knot.

TIP

If your hair is freshly washed, it can easily slip out of your fingers. I'd suggest using a little hairspray to give it some "grip" so it will stay in place.

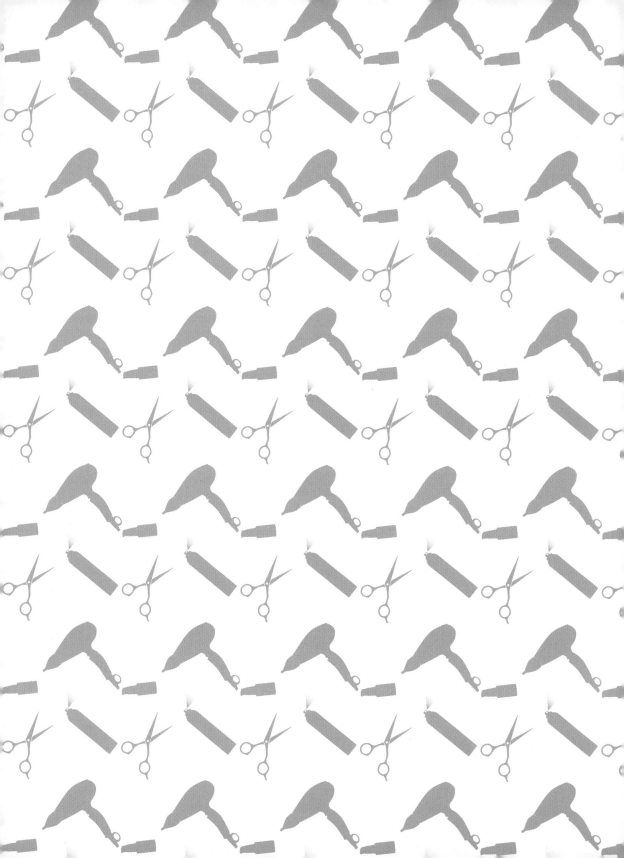

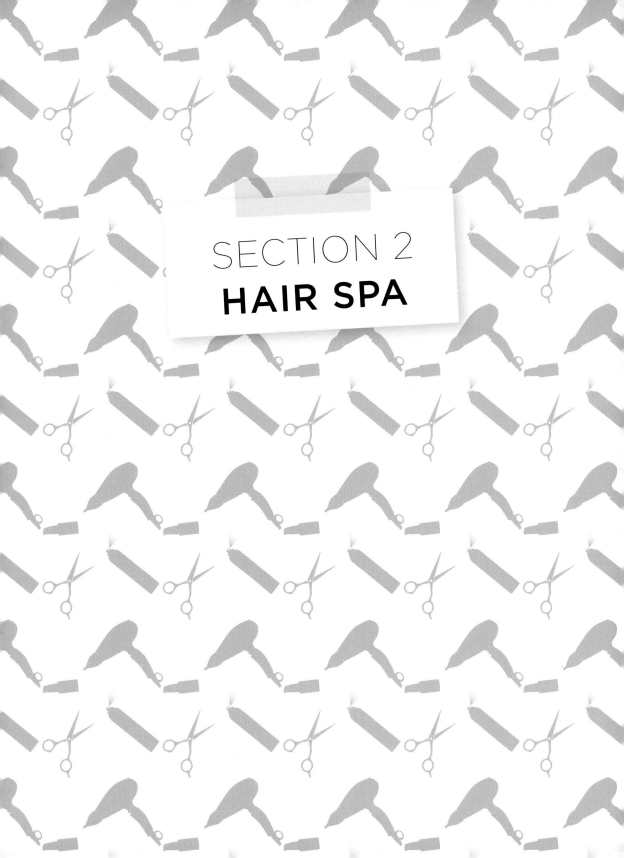

SECTION 2
HAIR SPA

CHAPTER 6
PROBLEMS & SOLUTIONS

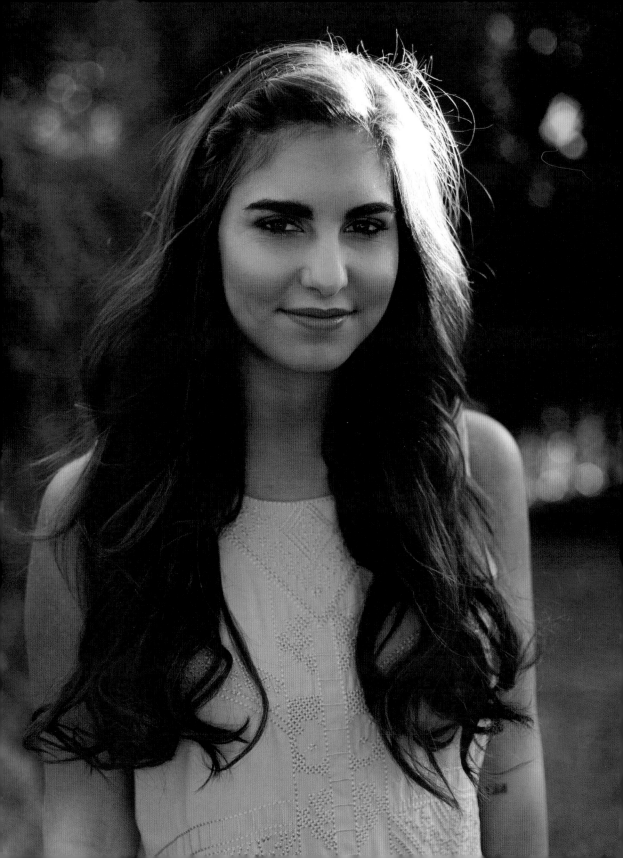

HAIR-CARE BASICS

By following these hair-care basics, you will have the healthy hair you crave so you can achieve gorgeous styles. Here are a few of my best tips.

SHAMPOO AND CONDITIONER

Use the appropriate shampoo and conditioner for your hair type. All hair-product bottles state which hair type they suit, so always check before you buy. If you still aren't sure, ask your hairstylist.

Shampoo as required. If your hair isn't greasy or dirty, then avoid over-shampooing your hair. Most importantly, avoid shampooing your hair on a daily basis because you will strip your hair of the natural oils secreted by your scalp that help moisturize and condition your hair. Well-moisturized hair will look awesome in your updos or braids. Use conditioner from the mid-shaft of the hair to the ends to prevent greasiness and avoid conditioning the roots, which will weigh your hair down.

TRIMS

To maintain the best hair possible, have your hair trimmed regularly. I usually recommend that pixie-length hair should be trimmed every four to six weeks and mid-length to long hair every six to eight weeks. This will help you eliminate split ends before they get out of control.

BRUSHING

Make sure to brush your hair at least once a day. This will stimulate your scalp, allowing the hair follicles to grow. You need to be tangle free to create your hairstyles.

KEEP UP ON COLOR

If you choose to color your hair, make sure to keep up on it. There is nothing worse than a gorgeous updo with some horrible roots.

If you have your hair colored with an all-over basic color, make sure to get your roots touched up every four to six weeks. If you have highlights, I suggest redoing them every eight to ten weeks.

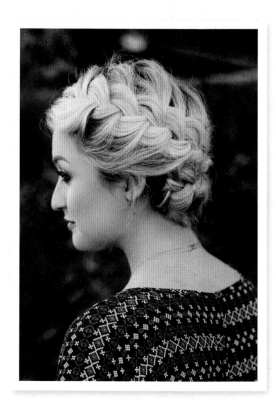

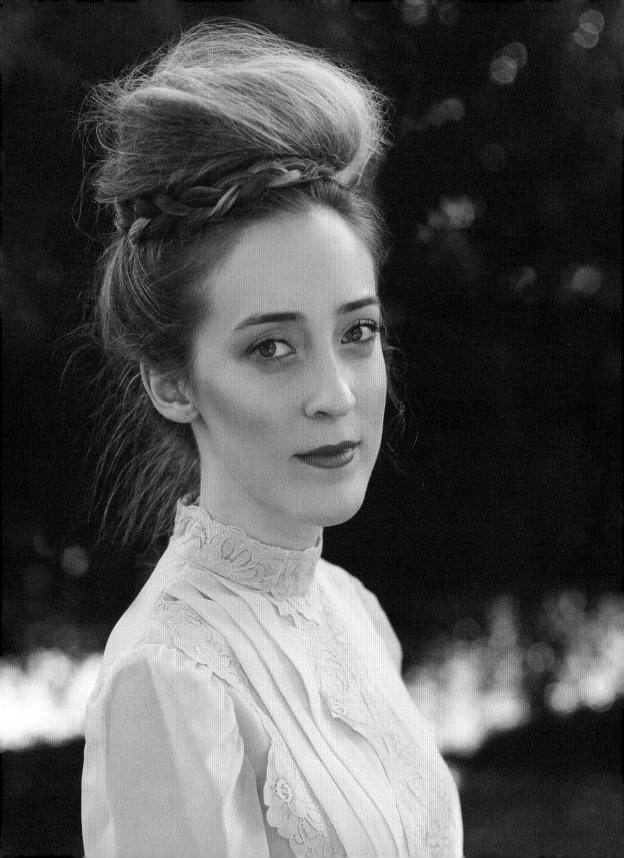

FINE AND OILY HAIR

If you have fine or oily hair, read this section to identify which products you can use to achieve the best results when attempting any type of upstyle, braid, bun, or twist.

FINE HAIR

Fine hair suits most updos or hairstyles but it is helpful to use volumizing products and texturizers to add body.

Before you dry your hair, use a mousse, spray gel, or root booster to add volume and texture to the roots. These products help plump up the hair. Blow dry from the opposite direction to which the hair lies for lift and volume at the roots.

Styles that are hard to achieve with fine-textured hair are braided hairstyles and upstyles that require a lot of volume.

NORMAL TO OILY HAIR

Normal to oily hair textures are ideal for upstyles, twists, and braids. Typically, normal hair textures are a bit fuller than fine textures, allowing the hairstyle to have more volume, curl easier, and stay in place better.

If your hair is normal to oily, opt for shampoos appropriate for your hair type that lather well. They will give your hair some bounce. You should be able to use all types of hair products, including hair conditioners.

OILY HAIR

If your hair is extremely oily, you may find it hard to prevent your hairstyle from falling flat. Simply add some dry shampoo and/or hair powder at the roots to help give a matte finish with plenty of volume.

You should avoid using silkening cremes or any oil-based conditioning products close to the scalp because they will add to the oiliness of your hair. Use lightweight conditioner.

After your shower, apply a leave-in conditioner, then your styling products, such as root lifters, which combat oiliness. Blow dry as you prefer.

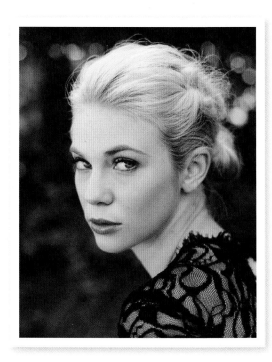

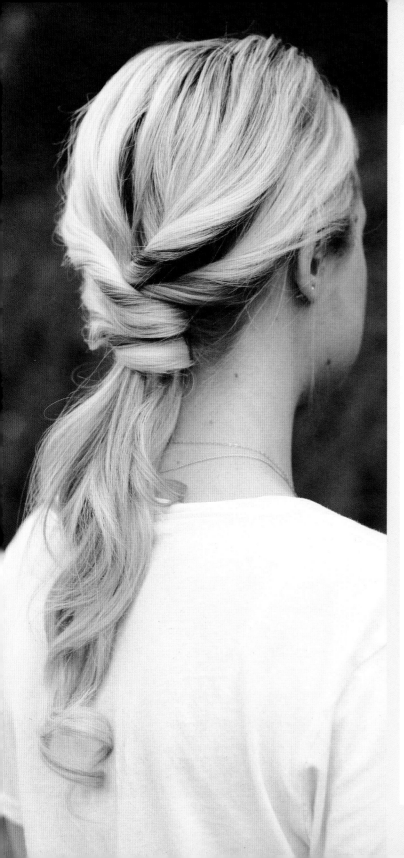

FINE HAIR PRODUCTS

- Use a lightweight shampoo and conditioner. A heavy moisturizing product will weigh down your hair and make it oily.

- After a shower, apply a lightweight leave-in conditioner, then apply a root lifter or texturizer.

- Use flexible-hold hairspray, and try shine spray to add texture and shine.

- On second-day hair you can use a dry shampoo to add volume. If you have oily hair, this will give a matte finish.

- Avoid oils, heavy serums, waxes, and pomades.

NORMAL AND OILY HAIR PRODUCTS

- Use a cleansing shampoo and lightweight conditioner.

- Use a mousse or root lifter when blow drying and styling; they contain alcohol, which will soak up oil.

- Use a medium-hold hairspray and dry shampoo on first- and second-day hair to help create bulk and soak up excess oils.

FRIZZY AND DRY HAIR

If you have frizzy hair, you can wear most hairstyles such as twists, upstyles, and top knots. For some styles, especially when wearing your hair down, you may want to pre-straighten your hair a little to eliminate the frizz. If you're creating a braided style, it will be hard to see the definition in the braid if your hair is very frizzy.

FRIZZY HAIR

Straight or sleek styles are difficult to create successfully with frizzy hair. You can easily straighten your hair yourself by using my straight hair tutorial (see page 42) and using the right oil-based products to help combat the frizz.

Use shampoos and styling aids that add moisture and seal the hair cuticle. Look for a moisturizing shampoo and conditioner that are suitable for frizzy hair. You can also buy curl amplifiers and oil-based products (see page 166).

DRY HAIR

Believe it or not, dry hair that has been chemically processed can be the best hair for creating updos, twists, and braids. This is because the hair cuticle has been broken down by chemicals, which makes the hair more pliable and creates the necessary texture to hold styles well.

Styles that don't work well for dry hair are sleeker looks because you may have some breakage and flyaways. But you can add some silkening cremes to fight the flyaways and fix the dry ends.

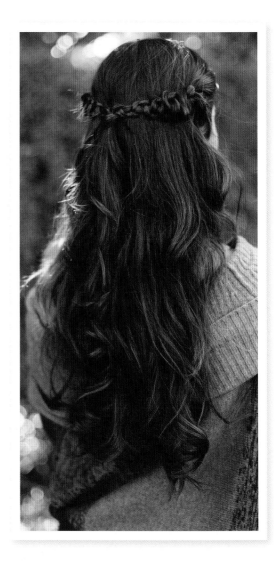

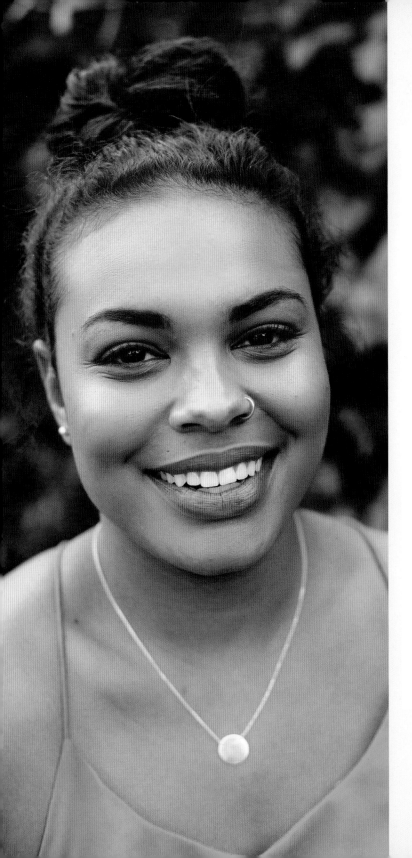

WASHING TIPS FOR FRIZZY AND DRY HAIR

- It is best not to wash your hair too frequently. Sometimes, you can get away with not shampooing your hair in the shower but just using conditioner. Your natural oils and the conditioner will help calm the frizziness.

- Before you wash your hair, add an oil-based serum or coconut oil to your hair from mid-shaft to ends. This adds an extra layer of protection to prevent oils being stripped out of the hair when shampooing. It's important to only shampoo the roots and not the ends, where hair tends to be drier and have more frizz.

- In the shower, use a wide-toothed comb to gently comb your hair after conditioning it. After your shower, lightly towel dry your hair, then use an oil-based product from roots to ends before styling.

FLAT HAIR

Some types of hair can be flat and limp, such as silky, heavy hair; fine hair that lacks volume; and coarse, thick hair. However, there are several low-volume styles that work beautifully for flat hair and some hairstyles that require a bit of teasing at the roots, which will help transform flat locks into beautiful bouncy tresses.

PRODUCTS

Use a volumizing shampoo and conditioner; they tend not to be heavy and leave your hair with extra bounce. I also recommend using root lifters, volumizing gels, and mousses before blow drying. After blow drying, use hair powders or dry texturizers, which will give your hair the fullness that it lacks naturally.

BLOW DRYING

Blow drying your hair the right way is the key to improving flat, limp hair. Make sure to blow dry your hair the opposite way to how it lies because this will help create long-lasting volume at the roots. Once the hair is 90 percent dry, I suggest going in with a round brush and working on lifting the roots area while blow drying at the same time.

CHEMICAL TEXTURE

Chemical texture is created when you color your hair and it helps break down the cuticle. If your hair is really heavy, silky, or fine, having a color service will help rough up the cuticle, giving your hair a bit more height. You don't need to go overboard—a few highlights on top or an all-over color will give some extra life to your hair.

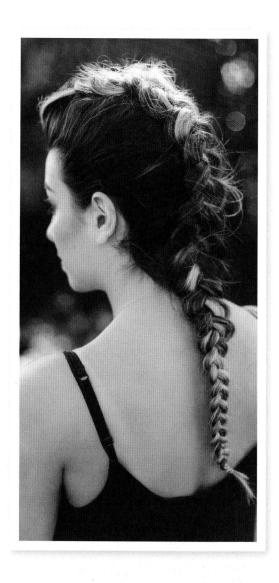

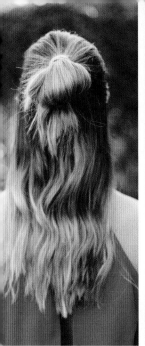

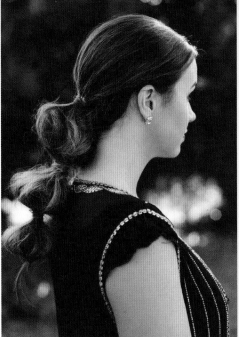

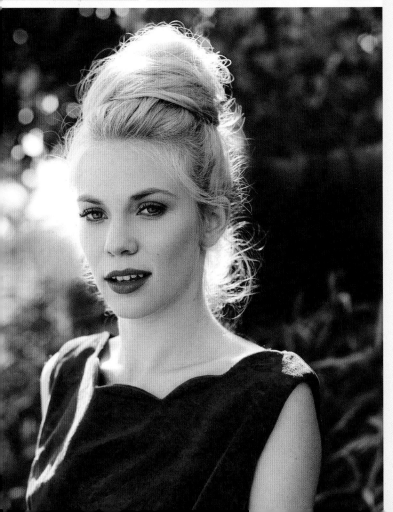

VOLUME

- If your flat hair lacks movement, adding a few layers on the top will give it more volume because it won't be so weighed down, and it will give your hair more movement.

- To create lots of volume with second-day hair, add a few curls with a curling iron on top of your head and pin them into place with a pin-curl clip until they cool down. This will help create fullness at the roots that will last all day.

- Wear the top-knot hairstyle to provide lots of volume on top of your head (see page 18). Before creating your top knot, add hair powder to create a fuller texture.

THICK HAIR

It seems we always want what we don't have. Fine-haired ladies want thick hair and thick-haired ladies crave less hair. Thick hair can be quite challenging due to its bulkiness and heaviness but there are several ways to wrangle thick locks.

LAYERS

Having the right haircut is important. If you have extremely thick hair, I recommend thinning the hair out a little to reduce the bulk. By introducing layers, you will create more movement throughout the hair, making it easier to manage on a daily basis.

ROOT LIFTERS

If your hair is really thick, it can sometimes become flat. Add a root lifter before blow drying to provide volume at the roots.

RECOMMENDED STYLES

Good hairstyles for thick hair include straight hair, braids, and low-volume upstyles. Straight hair (see page 42) hangs straight and flat to the head, and braids such as the French braid and the five-strand braid (see pages 80 and 146) are fuller and more dramatic on thick hair. Low-volume upstyles involve putting just some of your hair up, such as the half-down looped pony, the woven pony, and the flower bun (see pages 14, 84, and 100).

TOOLS

You don't want to skimp on the tools when dealing with thick hair. It can take a long time to blow dry and I recommend a good-quality dryer, which can cut down your drying time by half. Opt for an ionic blow dryer, which will help dry your hair cuticle from the inside out. When styling, use sectioning clips to take small sections.

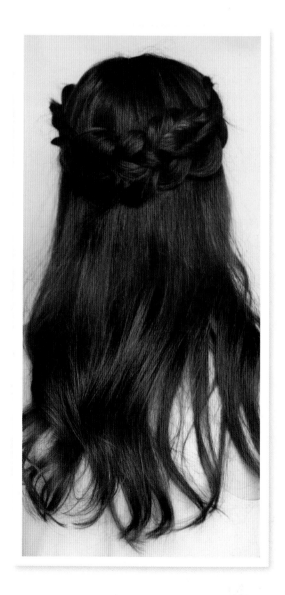

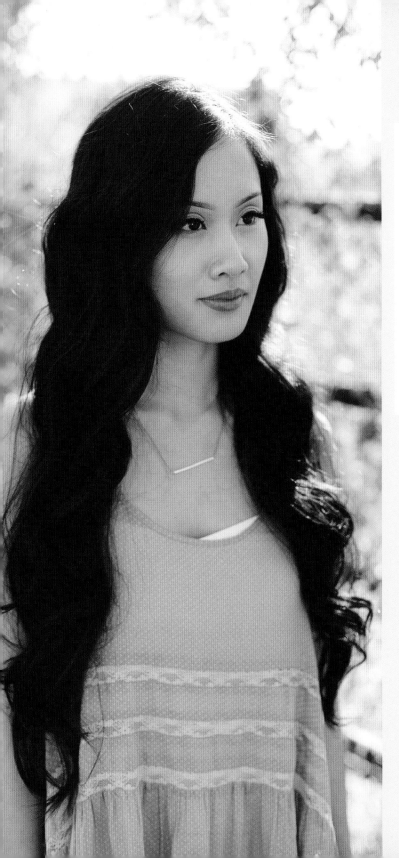

HIDING BULK

- If you are trying to hide bulk inside an updo, you can braid thick hair tight to the hair scalp and create an upstyle on top of it to reduce the volume.

- If your hair is really thick and you want a "barely there" wave, try using a flat-iron wave technique as on page 60, which will help flatten your thick hair.

HAIR PRODUCTS

Understanding hair products can be overwhelming, especially when there are so many out there in the market. Once you have a good understanding of your basic hair type, work out which products are suitable for you and which are best avoided.

DRY SHAMPOOS

In many of the hair tutorials, I mention using dry shampoo. A dry shampoo isn't a shampoo at all but is intended to be used on second-day hair. It is an aerosol spray bottle that you hold about 6–8 in (15–20 cm) away from your hair while spraying the matte-like powder all over. The powder helps soak up any excess oils from your hair. If your hair is normally oily, you can use it after you've washed and blow dried your hair as a precautionary measure. It also helps create bulk on fine hair.

SILKENING CREMES

Silkening cremes are used for hair that is dry, porous, and tends to have a bit of frizz. These cremes help smooth bothersome flyaways down in a matter of minutes and add softness as well as shine. Depending on the density of your hair, use one to three large dollops of creme and spread it through your hair after shampooing, conditioning, and towel drying. Work the product from mid-shaft down to the ends. Avoid using it at the roots because this can create greasiness or an oily appearance.

ELIXIRS OR OILS

There are several different types of oils so it can be hard to find the right one. I usually look for a product that contains argan, Moroccan, or sesame oil. Always check the recommended hair types on the bottle and buy according to your hair type. Elixirs or oils are usually used for shine, frizz control, and moisturizing.

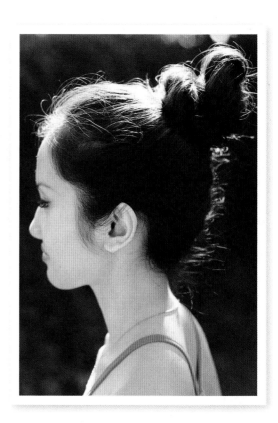

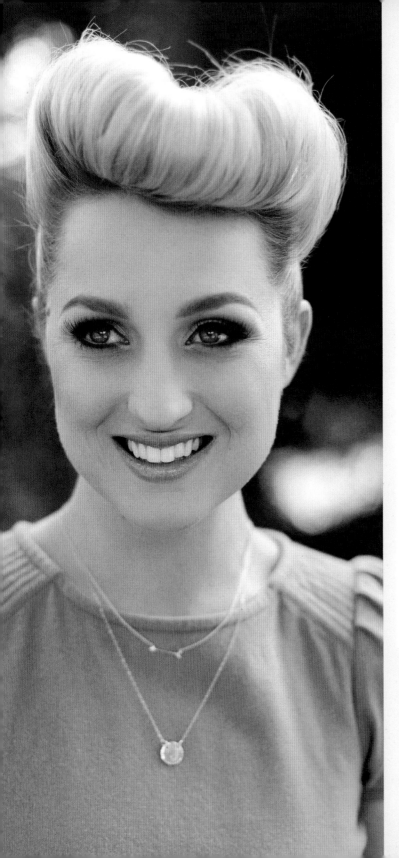

HAIRSPRAYS

Did you know that you can achieve different types of holds with different hairsprays? Hairspray holds range from flexible, medium, and workable to hard-hold, and some even come with a bit of shine.

- Flexible spray gives some hold while allowing the hair to have some movement, so it's good for down styles.
- Medium spray has a light to medium hold that can be used while curling hair.
- Workable spray is used frequently during up styling because it allows you to manipulate the hair into place.
- Firm hold is the hairspray for finishing if you want your hair to stay in place all day and is great for updos.

HAIR PRODUCTS

USING OILS

Make sure you use your oil properly. Usually a pump or two should be plenty. I recommend using it after you have showered and towel dried your hair—apply it from a couple of inches away from your roots down to your ends. If your hair is still a bit frizzy or not as shiny as you would like, add a small amount to your hair when it's dry. You can even use it again the following day to help freshen your hair and smooth any pesky flyaways. If your hair is particularly dry, try applying some of your oil-based product before you shampoo and condition your hair. This will act as a hair protectant to help lock in the natural oils so that the shampoo doesn't strip them away.

HAIR POWDERS/MICRO DUSTS

Hair powders (also known as micro dusts) are a fairly new product that you can use directly on the scalp for volume and lift. I call it "backcombing in a bottle" because you take small sections at the root area where you want the lift, sprinkle a little powder there, and you immediately get roots that are full of volume. These products work well for ladies who want volume that will last all day, whether in down styles or updos.

MOUSSES

I recommend using mousse on hair that is fine, curl resistant, or lacking in volume. Apply a large dollop on towel-dried hair from the roots to the ends and then blow dry.

ROOT LIFTERS

A root lifter is great for women who lack volume at the roots because their hair is fine, or it's thick and heavy. Comb your hair directly back and where it naturally splits, aggressively add your root lifter on the roots. Then blow dry your hair the opposite way the hair is going to lie in order to achieve lots of volume.

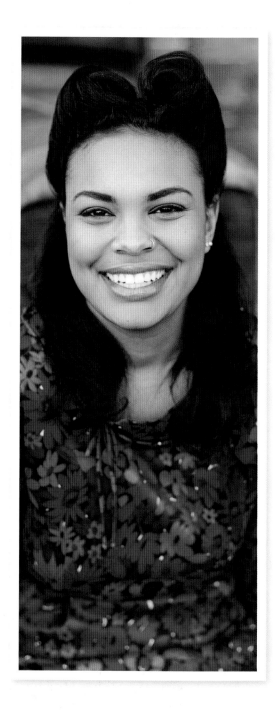

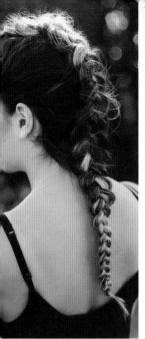

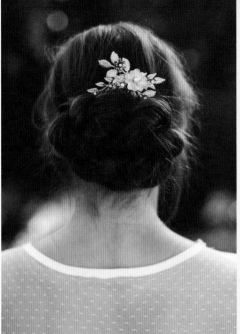

HAIRSPRAY—OTHER USES

- If your bobby pins tend to slip out of your hair, try spraying them with a bit of hairspray before using them. The hairspray will add grip.

- If your hair is prone to static, use some hairspray and then the back of your comb to help press down unwanted flyaways.

SHINE SPRAYS

If your hair lacks luster, use a shine spray once you have completed your style. Shine sprays work well on updos and hair that has been recently blown out with a round brush. Hold the can 6–8 in (15–20 cm) away from your scalp and apply all over.

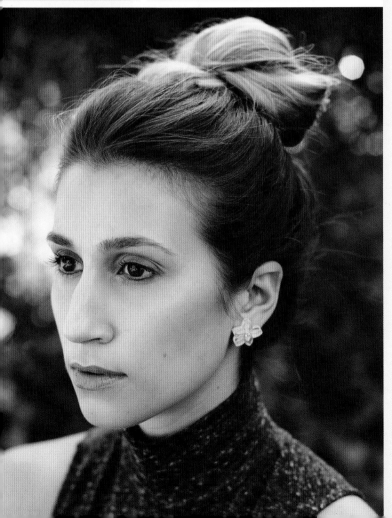

DOS AND DON'TS

When you're creating fun hairstyles, make sure you're aware of the important dos and don'ts. Here are a few of my favorites.

DOS:

DIRTY HAIR

This is not a myth, friends! Dirty hair is a major plus when it comes to up styling and braids. If you start with day-old hair when creating an upstyle, your scalp's natural oils will help give your hair some added shine as well as smooth down any unwanted flyaways. It is also easier to create braids when your hair is dirty—you are less likely to end up with pesky pieces sticking straight out because the natural oils in your hair provide added weight and allow it to lie smooth.

USE HEAT PROTECTANT

Some women think they can get away without using a heat protectant when curling or flat ironing their hair. But this really is necessary if you want to maintain the integrity of your hair. Heat protectants are essential to protect your hair from heat damage. Follow the instructions on the back of the bottle for optimum results.

USE THE RECOMMENDED HAIR PRODUCTS

Make sure to always use the recommended hair product for the style. You may want to be natural and not use hair products, but if you want the best results when creating certain styles, I highly recommend using the hair products suggested.

DON'TS:

SKIP BRUSHING

Don't skip brushing your hair before creating your hairstyle. When you start knot-free, it will enable you to take clean sections and prevent your hair from tangling while you work on the style. Always start brushing from the ends and work toward the roots.

NEGLECT A HAIRCUT

Friends, getting a haircut on a regular basis is hugely beneficial. Not only will your hair grow faster because you get rid of split ends, but also your upstyles and braids will look a hundred times better with healthy ends.

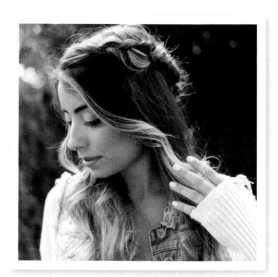

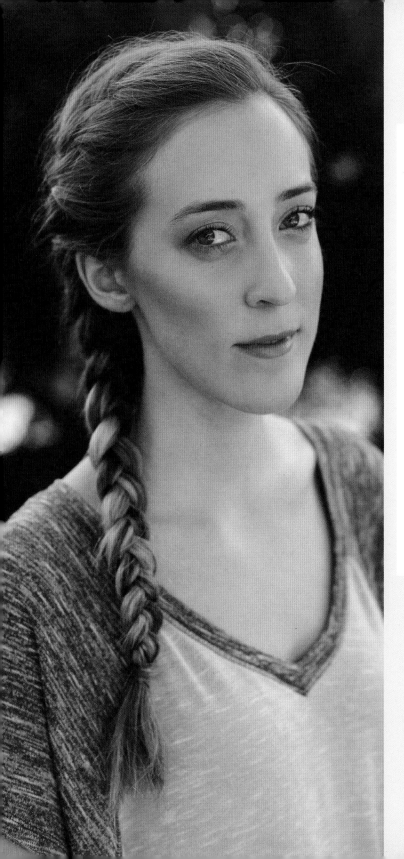

USING HOT TOOLS

One of the biggest mistakes my clients make is using hot tools when their hair is not completely dry.

- If you use an iron on your hair while it has moisture in it, you will damage the hair, leaving it feeling dry and possibly frying the ends.

- When you want to use any hot tool, such as a flat iron, curling iron, or hot rollers, always feel your hair first. If your hair is cool to the touch, there is still some moisture in the hair. Wait until your hair is warm to the touch before you use your hot tools.

COLORING ADVICE

Whether you color your hair in the comfort of your own home or get it done at the hair salon, it's important to know how to take care of your newly colored locks. Here are a few basic tips to help you get the most out of your fresh look.

KEEP WASHING TO A MINIMUM

I recommend that you wash your colored hair as little as possible. Every time you wash it, you risk the vibrancy fading a bit, so it's best not to wash your hair every day if possible.

FIND THE RIGHT SHAMPOO

If you have just received a color service such as a highlight and/or all-over color, make sure you maintain your locks with the correct kind of shampoos and conditioners. For all-over colored hair, opt for a shampoo that is color safe and sulfate free. Most bottles will state on the label that the product is geared toward highlighted or colored hair, but be sure to ask your stylist if you are unable to find a suitable one.

WASH WITH COOL WATER

It's not just a question of having the right shampoo. If you want the vibrancy of your color to last as long as possible, I suggest using lukewarm to cool water when shampooing and conditioning. Hot water will open up the hair cuticle, allowing color molecules to escape, but if you use cool water, those molecules will stay there longer. Also, cool water lays down the hair cuticle, reflecting light and giving a shiny appearance.

USE LEAVE-IN CONDITIONER

If your hair has been highlighted and your stylist has used a lightener, it can leave your hair feeling rather dry. After you shower, I recommend using a leave-in conditioner with UV protection, which will provide extra moisture and reduce color fading.

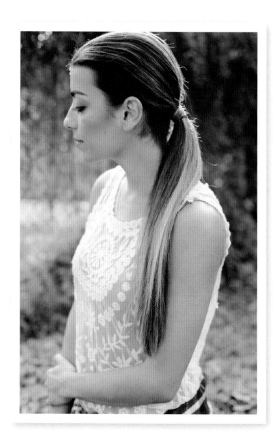

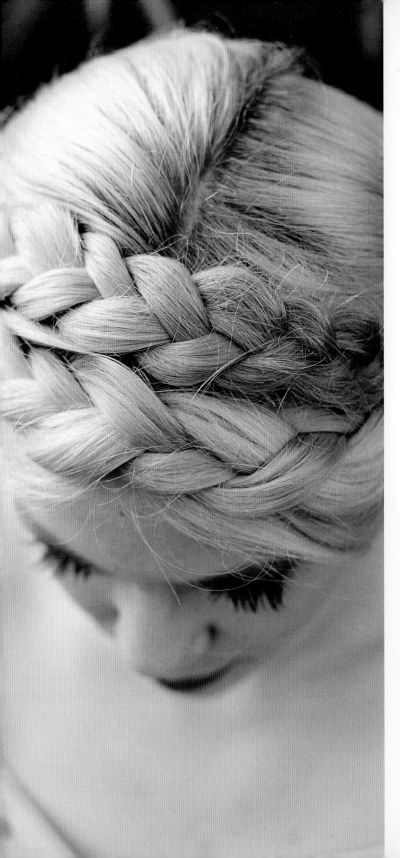

SUN PROTECTION

If your hair has been colored, it's best to protect it from the sun, especially in the hot summer months:

- Find a leave-in conditioner that contains UV protectant. This protects the hair against unwanted fading.

- If you find yourself in a situation with no sun-protection products, you can grab a scarf, hat, or a cute bandana to cover your hair when heading outdoors so that the sun doesn't take a toll on your freshly colored locks.

HEALTHY HAIR

Achieving healthy hair can be difficult if you don't have a treatment program to follow. Just use my basic tips and you will have your friends begging you to find out what you did differently to achieve such luscious locks.

HAIR MASKS

There are many elements that can wreak havoc on our locks, so treat your hair by using a hair mask. If your hair is extremely dry, I suggest using a mask once a week. If it is a little dry or unruly, do it every other week. Using a mask regularly will help to condition and strengthen your hair (see page 177).

EAT WELL

Eating a well balanced diet will help provide the essential vitamins your hair needs. Make sure you eat plenty of proteins; your hair and skin are made out of protein and these provide the basis for strong hair. You should also eat foods rich in omega 3 oils. If your diet is deficient in these oils, you are liable to suffer from a dry scalp and dull hair. Eat your way to lustrous hair by eating salmon, walnuts, flaxseeds, and sardines.

HYDRATE

Drink lots of water to help hydrate your hair. If you're dehydrated, your skin and hair will be as well. Make sure to drink at least the recommended amount of water each day.

GIVE YOUR HAIR A BREAK

If you have a week when your hair is feeling dry, avoid styles requiring a blow dryer or curling iron and opt for top knots, braids, or ponytails.

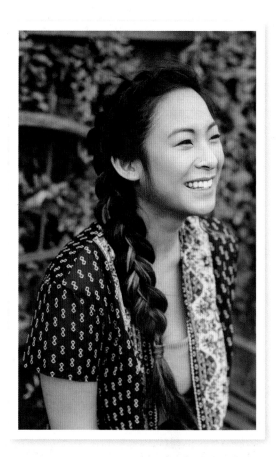

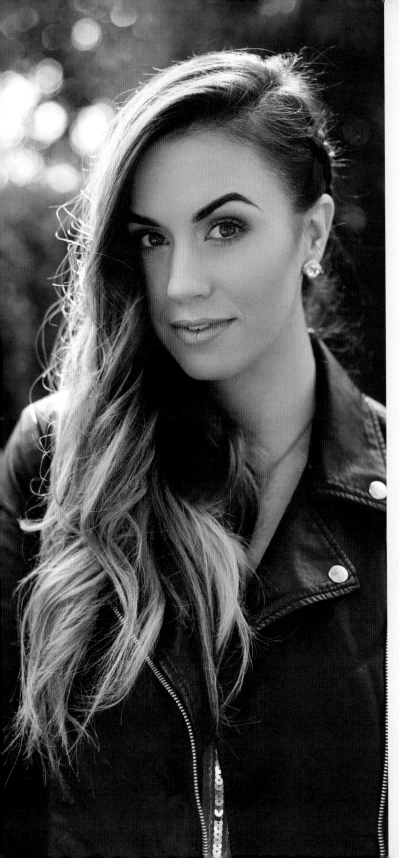

VITAMIN SUPPLEMENTS

The best way to obtain vitamins is from your diet. But if you are unable to eat enough vitamin-rich foods, consider taking vitamins that help to maintain healthy locks. Usually the bottle will state it is for maintaining healthy hair and promoting hair growth. Vitamins C and B are suitable as these help to prevent dry hair and split ends, but always discuss this with your doctor first, if needed.

NATURAL REMEDIES

Calling all of my ladies who like to do things the natural way! Did you know that you can reach into your pantry and prepare natural hair-care remedies quickly and easily in the comfort of your own home? Here are my top three natural hair-care treatments.

EGGS

Repair your hair instantly by reaching into your fridge and grabbing some eggs. Not only do eggs have tons of protein that is great for strengthening your hair, but also the yolk is packed with nutrients that will leave your locks nourished and moisturized. For this treatment, mix two egg yolks with two tablespoons of olive oil and then dilute the mixture with a little water. After you shampoo, apply the treatment all over your hair as you would a hair mask and let it soak in for 15 to 20 minutes before washing out. Then use your normal daily conditioner and rinse. I recommend doing this treatment a couple of times a month to nourish your hair.

BEER (REALLY!)

Flat, limp hair is a common problem. If you're in a lifeless hair rut you can easily make your locks voluminous by grabbing a beer. The hops and yeast in beer help create volume and add texture to the hair. Use a light beer at room temperature and pour it over your hair after you shampoo. Rinse and style as normal. Skip on your conditioner because it will weigh down your new lifted locks.

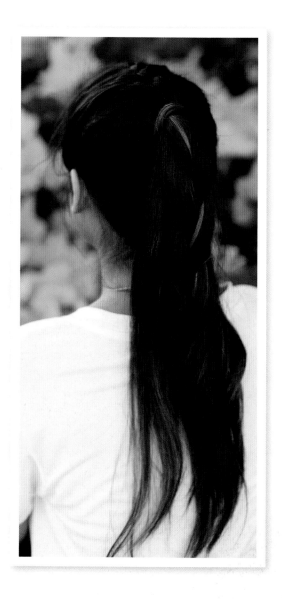

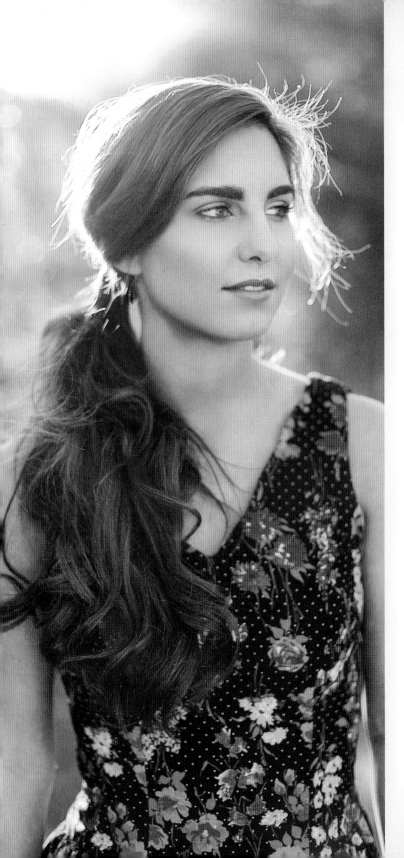

COCONUT OIL

We all have days where our hair could use a bit more shine, and coconut oil is great for this: it's extremely moisturizing and provides nutrients. You can use the coconut oil in several ways, but I prefer it as a mask or used directly on the hair.

• To use as a hair mask, use coconut oil in the shower after you have shampooed your hair. Warm and soften 1–2 tablespoons of coconut oil in your hands by rubbing it in your palms. Apply the oil from the mid shaft down to the ends. Let it soak in and do its magic for a few minutes and rinse away. Your hair should be instantly shiny and smell divine.

• You can also use coconut oil instead of a shine serum once you have dried your hair. Simply dab your finger in the oil (a little goes a long way) and rub it in your hands to warm it. Apply from a couple of inches away from the roots to the ends. This will help tame any flyaways as well as instantly giving your hair some shine.

TREATING PROBLEM HAIR

Problem hair includes sleek, thick hair that is too slippery for braids or curls, chemically treated hair that has been over-processed, and frizzy, coarse hair. With these types of hair, it can be quite difficult to achieve fun braids or updos, but there are a few tricks, tips, and products that will allow you to achieve the looks you have been dying to try.

SLEEK HAIR

Sleek hair that is too slippery for braids or curls can be problematic when you want a soft updo or a large statement braid. The problem is that this type of hair is too healthy. Yes, I said too healthy! Although sleek hair looks beautiful, the texture needs to be roughed up a bit so that it can hold curls and braids and stay in upstyles.

After you wash your hair, apply a mousse or a spray gel, which will give the hair more grip, texture, and hold. Once you have blow dried your hair, try curling it, and it should hold much better. You can also apply a bit of dry shampoo when braiding sleek hair, which will coarsen the texture and allow it to stay full rather than going flat.

DRY AND CHEMICALLY TEXTURED HAIR

Chemically textured hair can be troublesome owing to unwanted breakage that will create broken pieces and flyaways in your styles. Take care of chemically textured hair by adding moisture to it with products such as deep conditioners, silkening cremes, and hair-repair products. If you're creating a style and you have an unruly breakage, add a little silkening creme to that area to help smooth the ends.

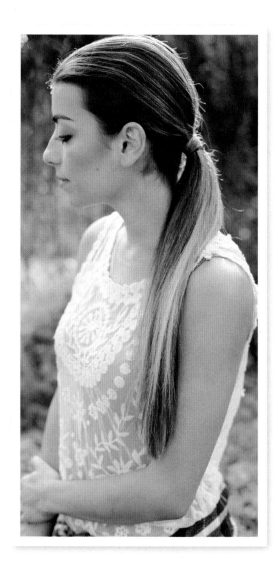

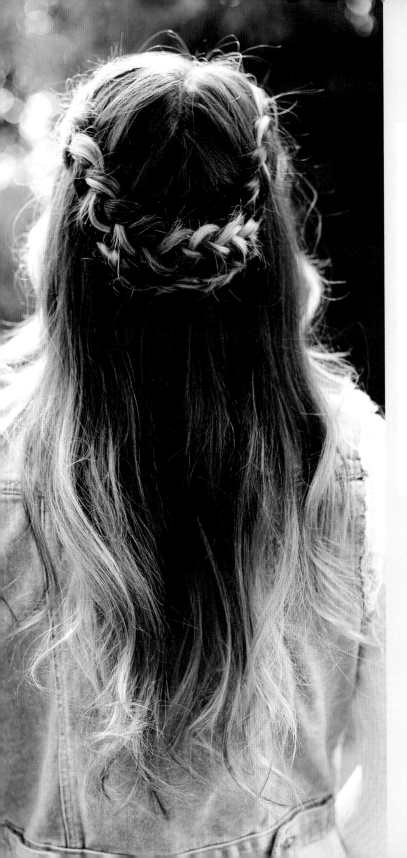

FRIZZY HAIR

Frizzy and coarse hair can be a real pain to deal with if you want to go for a smooth look. These tips can help:

- Try using an oil-based elixir or a silkening creme and blow dry your hair straight down with the nozzle parallel to the hairbrush. This will help smooth down unwanted flyaways.
- Use hair masks on a regular basis to add moisture to the hair and smooth down unwanted frizz (see page 177).

TOOLS

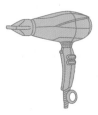

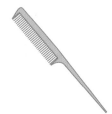

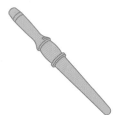

BLOW DRYER WITH NOZZLE

A blow dryer with a nozzle is a must-have. Opt for a professional ionic blow dryer with a powerful motor, which will cut drying time in half.

WEAVING COMB

Also known as a rat-tail comb or tail comb. This type of comb has a fine-toothed side and a narrow end made of plastic or metal. A tail comb is great for taking perfect sections, and hairstylists use it while coloring hair.

CURLING WAND

Also known as a clampless iron, this has a barrel that you wrap your hair around while using gloves to protect your hands from the heat. This type of tool produces wavy curls.

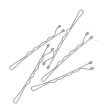

WIDE-TOOTHED COMB

The best comb to use for thick and frizzy hair; it is gentle on the hair, creating less friction yet detangling hair effectively.

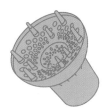

BOBBY PINS

Bobby pins are used during upstyling or braiding. They are designed to help your style stay in place. Always use bobby pins that match your hair coloring so that they blend in.

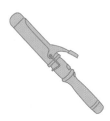

DIFFUSER

This tool is for people with wavy or curly hair. It's an attachment that you put on the end of your blow dryer to protect your hair from direct heat, and it allows you to scrunch up your hair as you dry to give a natural look with minimal frizz.

CURLING IRON

This is a styling tool that becomes hot and is designed to help create waves and curls in your hair. The clamp allows you to hold on to your hair as you ease it through the hair tong. Many curling irons have an adjustable heat setting to suit all different hair types.

COMB

The wide-toothed side is best for combing thick and wet hair, while the fine-toothed side is great for sleeker styles.

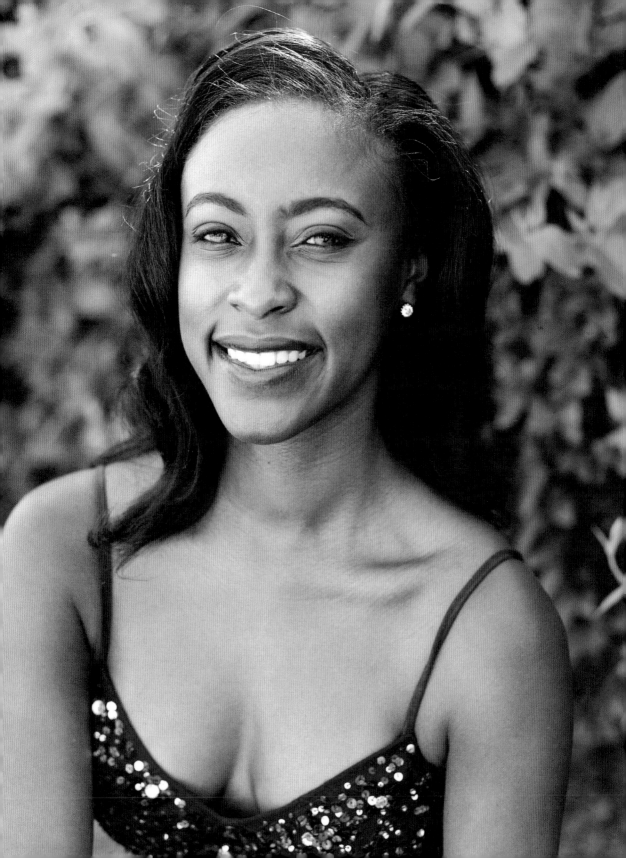

TOOLS

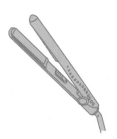

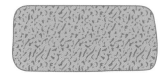

HAIR PADDING
Synthetic padding used to add height and volume to upstyles.

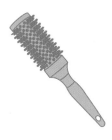

FLAT IRON
Also known as a straightening iron, this is a hot styling tool with two flat plates that press your hair together to create a smooth, straight appearance.

ROUND BRUSH
Round brushes are used during blow drying for volume and smoothness and to create some bend at the ends of your hair. For volume, wrap the hair around the round brush, placing it close to the roots, and hold in position while using your dryer. Allow your hair to cool before releasing the brush.

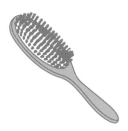

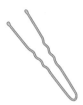

PADDLE BRUSH
This is a flat brush most commonly used in detangling when the hair is wet but it can also be used during blow drying for low-volume styles.

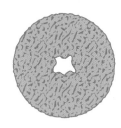

FRINGE PIN
These pins are great for chignons, twists, and buns. When using them simply squeeze them slightly as you insert them into your style, so that when you release them they hold their

PIN-CURL CLIP
This clip is used to keep hair in place while you are forming your upstyle or you can use it to help mold a curl while it sets.

SOCK-BUN DONUT
This is hair padding most commonly used for the sock-bun hairstyle. It works well for ladies with fine hair who want to make their hair appear thicker and fuller.

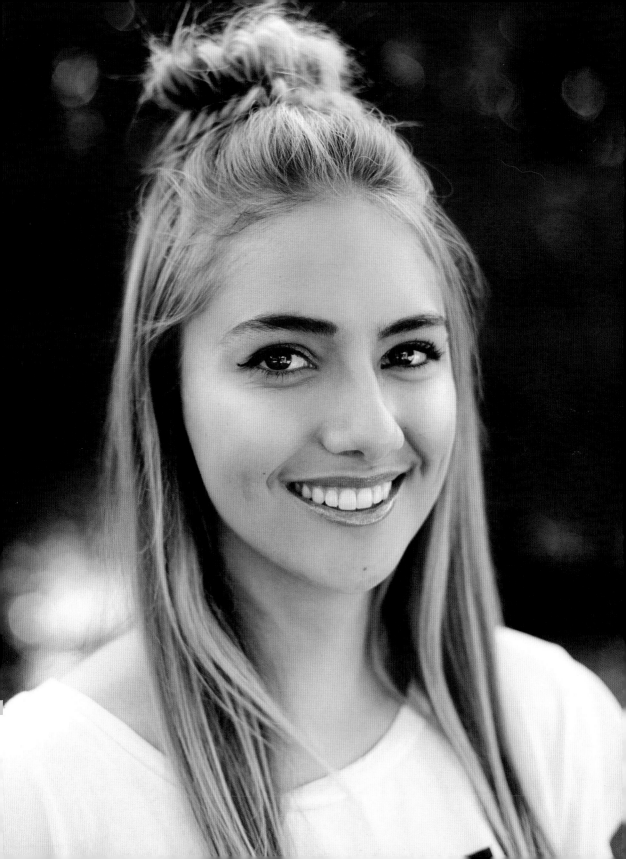

GLOSSARY

BACKCOMB

This technique, also known as teasing, involves using a comb or brush to create bulk and volume at the roots. You take a small section of hair, hold it straight up, and aggressively move your comb or brush downward toward the scalp.

BLOW DRYING

This is a technique where you blow dry the hair from towel dried to 100 percent dry by using a blow dryer and a brush such as a round brush or paddle brush.

BRAID

Also referred to as a plait, a technique that involves weaving sections of hair into each other. There are several ways you can braid your hair, including three-strand braids, French braids, and fishtail braids.

CHIGNON

This is a classic bun shape that usually sits around the nape of the neck.

CROWN

The area on the top and center of the head where your skull naturally starts curving down.

CURL CREAM/AMPLIFIER

Curl cream or amplifier controls frizziness and holds curls in place.

CURLING IRON

A hot styling tool used to create curls and waves. There are several sizes ranging from 1/4 in (6 mm) to 2 in (5 cm).

DRY SHAMPOO

A hair styling product that helps give greasy or second-day hair look freshly washed. It's also a good product for adding texture to hair before styling.

DUCK-BILL CLIP

Long, slim clip used for holding the hair during styling.

FLAT IRON

Also known as a straightening iron, this is a styling tool that gets hot so that you can straighten your hair in seconds or tame unwanted frizz and flyaways. You can also use it to add loose curls.

HAIR ELASTIC

Also known as a hair band, elastic band or a hair tie, hair elastics are used to tie up hair.

HAIR EXTENSION

Synthetic or real human hair woven together on a hair weft that you can attach to your own natural hair to add length or volume. There are several different types of extensions for temporary use that can be attached using glue or tape, protein bonded or clipped in.

HAIRLINE

This is the hair that grows along the perimeter of your head, including around your face and ears and along your neckline.

HAIR MIST

Anti-frizz in a bottle: it makes dry hair soft and shiny.

HAIR POWDER / MICRO DUST

A light styling powder used at the roots to add volume and lift.

HAIR TEXTURE

A term used to classify the type of hair you have depending on the curl pattern, volume, and consistency of your hair.

HAIR SECTION

A section of your hair that is clipped back while you work on other sections.

HAIR STRAIGHTENING SERUM

A product to protect your hair from heat damage and ease frizz when straightening.

HEAT PROTECTANT

A product to help protect hair when drying and straightening with hot tools.

MOUSSE

A light, fast-drying foam that gives extra volume, texture and shine. It can be used on wet or dry hair.

NAPE

The hair at the back of your neck.

SALT SPRAY

A product that pulls moisture and oils out of the hair, dries it, and coarsens the texture.

SHINE SERUM

A product to smooth the hair and enhance shine.

SHINE SPRAY

A spray for adding texture and shine to fine hair.

SPRAY GEL

A pump spray usually used on damp hair to shape or control waves or curls. It can be applied near the roots to add fullness and lift.

SPRAY WAX

A hairspray that add texture and definition and gives a tousled look.

CONTRIBUTORS

MODELS

Coley Arnold
Brooke Barker
Sakura Considine
Chelsea Cooper
Taylar Dickman
Alexandra Evjen
Lauren Garcia
Dorthy Ha
Bailey Harris
Jess Hause
Lindsey Holt
Angelica Karamooz
Candace Kim
Karra Labombarde
Marie McGrath
Bianca Mead
Alexis Mouer
Erika Naakka
Sungwook O Franke
Britnee Penson
Claire Planeta
Amanda Raye
Heather Rojo
Jessica Sarceda
Megan Tankeh
Amanda Shearer
Talina Talburt
Morgan Teresa
Mia Terezia
Arianna Theisen
Walker
Bella Wholey

HAIR

Christina Butcher
www.hairromance.com

Chelsea Cooper

Anthony Lunam
www.theorydesign.com

Tracy Melton
www.tracymeltonartistry.com

Missy Sue
www.missysue.com

Jay Olson
www.thebespokesalon.com

Amanda Raye
www.brokeandchic.com

Genevieve Reber
www.genevievereber.com

Jenny Strebe
www.theconfessionsofahairstylist
.com

Kyle Tuttle

Jamie Voelz
www.scussirsbeatpaper.com

Walker
www.walkerwerkshop.com

Demi Walsh
www.theoryhairdesign.com

Molly Gee Webster
www.mollygeedesigns.com

HAIR ACCESSORIES

Anna Catherine Photography
www.annacatherinephoto.com

Molly Gee Designs
www.mollygeedesigns.com

MAKEUP

Aeni Domme
www.aenidomme.com

Sandy Goldstein
www.sandyg.com

Kerri Metcalf
www.kerrimua.co

Stephanie Nault
www.stephanienault.com

Stephanie Neiheisel
www.snmakeupartist.com

Morgan Teresa
www.morganteresamakeup
.foliohd.com

PHOTOGRAPHY

Adam+Alli
www.adamplusalli.com

b. mo foto
http://bmofoto.com/blog/

Anna Catherine Photography
www.annacatherinephoto.com

Cassandra Eldridge
www.cassandraeldridge.com

Mary Costa Photography
www.marycostaphotography.com

Sarah Belgray
www.sarahbelgray.wordpress.com

Sara Bishop
www.sarabishop.com

Tiffany Egbert
www.tiffanyegbert.com

Laura Meek
http://laurameek.com

Sarah Nevels
www.talkstudiosphotography.
com

Danielle M. Sabol
www.daniellemsabol.com

Kym Ventola
www.ventolaphotography.com

WEBSITES

www.brokeandchic.com

www.brokemedia.com

www.junkinthetrunkvintage
apparel.com

www.missysue.com

www.of-north.com

www.sachastrebe.com

www.tremaineranch.com

BLOGGERS

Sakura Considine
www.somethingsakura.com

Alexandra Evjen
www.avestyles.com

Lauren Garcia
www.whatlolalikes.com

Candace Kim
www.candacevkim.com

Marie McGrath
www.thejoyoffashionblog.com

Claire Planeta
www.beautyandabargain.com

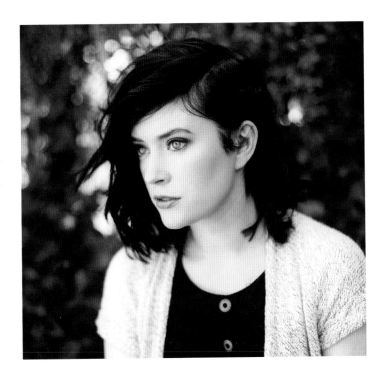

PHOTO CREDITS

Unless otherwise stated hair styling is by Jenny Strebe and photography is by Tiffany Egbert.

CHAPTER 1

page 14 Top: Makeup Aeni Domme; model Dorthy Ha. Bottom: Hair Walker; makeup Morgan Teresa; model Britnee Penson

page 16 Top: Makeup Aeni Domme; model Brooke Barker. Bottom left: Makeup Stephanie Neiheisel; photography Kaard Bombe; model Lauren Garcia. Below right: Photography Sara Nevels; model Alexandra Taylor

page 18 Top: Makeup Stephanie Neiheisel; model Lauren Garcia. Bottom: Hair and makeup Molly Gee Designs; photography Anna Catherine

page 20 Top: Hair and makeup Molly Gee Designs; photography Laura Meek. Bottom: Hair Anthony Lunam; makeup Stephanie Neiheisel; model Claire Planeta

page 22 Top: Photography Sara Nevels; model Sarah Hubbel. Bottom: Makeup Stephanie Neiheisel; model Jess Hause

page 24 Top: Makeup Aeni Domme; model Dorthy Ha. Bottom: Hair and makeup Molly Gee Designs; photography Anna Catherine Photography

page 26 Top: Hair Kyle Tuttle; makeup Morgan Teresa; model Sungwook O Franke. Bottom: Makeup Stephanie Neiheisel; model Alex Mouer

page 28 Top: Makeup Morgan Teresa; model Britnee Penson. Bottom left: Hair, makeup, and model Alexandra Evjen; photography Kym Ventola. Bottom right: Makeup Morgan Teresa; model Arianna Theisen

page 30 Top: Makeup Stephanie Neiheisel; model Jess Hause. Bottom: Hair and makeup Golden Locks; photography Mafalda Rodrigues; model Golden Locks. Bottom right: Hair Jay Olson; photography Sara Nevels; model Alexandra Taylor

page 32 Top: Makeup Stephanie Neiheisel; model Alex Mour. Bottom left: Makeup Stephanie Neiheisel; model Alex Mour. Bottom right: Makeup Morgan Teresa; model Sakura Considine

page 34 Top: Makeup Stephanie Neiheisel; model Claire Planeta. Bottom: Hair Jamie Voelz-Leaman; makeup Sandy Goldstein; model Ashley Lubich

page 36 Top: Hair and makeup Marie McGrath; photography and model Marie

McGrath. Bottom left: Makeup Morgan Teresa; model Morgan Teresa. Bottom right: Hair Walker; makeup Morgan Teresa; model Sungwook O Franke

page 38 Top: Hair Anthony Lunam; makeup Stephanie Neiheisel; model Jess Hause. Bottom: Hair Demi Walsh; makeup Stephanie Neiheisel; model Karra Labombarde

page 40 Top: Makeup Kerri Metcalf; model Talina Talburt, Bottom: Makeup Chante Fox; photography Sara Nevels; model Chante Fox

CHAPTER 2

page 44 Top: Makeup Stephanie Neiheisel; model Claire Planeta. Bottom: Hair Kyle Tuttle; makeup Morgan Teresa; model Sakura Considine

page 46 Top: Hair Demi Walsh; makeup Sandy Goldstein; model Bianca Mead. Bottom: Makeup Sandy Goldstein; model Taylar Dickman

page 48 Top: Hair Anthony Lunam; makeup Aeni Domme; model Angelica Karamooz. Bottom left: Makeup Stephanie Neiheisel; model Jessica Sarceda. Bottom right: Hair Walker; makeup Morgan Teresa; model Sungwook O Franke

page 50 Top: Hair and makeup Molly Gee Designs; photography Anna Catherine. Bottom left: Hair Hair Dreams; photography Maria Bradshaw. Bottom right: Hair and makeup Molly Gee Designs; photography Anna Catherine

page 52 Top: Makeup Stephanie Neiheisel; model Talina Talburt. Bottom: Hair Erika Naakka; photography Erika Naakka; model Erika Naakka

page 54 Top: Hair Demi Walsh; makeup Stephanie Neiheisel; model Talina Talburt. Bottom: Makeup Stephanie Neiheisel; model Jessica Sarceda

page 56 Top: Makeup Stephanie Neiheisel; model Jessica Sarceda. Bottom: Makeup Stephanie Neiheisel; model Courtney Larsen

page 58 Top: Makeup Stephanie Neiheisel; model Jess Hause. Bottom: Makeup Aeni Domme; model Anjelica Karamooz

page 60 Top: Hair Anthony Lunam; makeup Aeni Domme; model Lauren Garcia. Bottom left: Hair and makeup Molly Gee Designs; photography Anna Catherine. Bottom right: Hair Anthony Lunam; model Megan Tankeh

page 62 Top: Makeup Aeni Domme; model Megan Tankeh. Bottom: Makeup Anne Domme; model Dorthy Ha

page 64 Top: Makeup Stephanie Neiheisel; model Karra Labombarde. Bottom left: Makeup Stephanie Neiheisel; model Jessica Saceda. Bottom right: Hair Kyle Tuttle; makeup Morgan Teresa; model Sungwook O Franke

page 66 Top: Makeup Stephanie Neiheisel; model Claire Planeta. Bottom: Makeup Chelsea Cooper; model Chelsea Cooper

CHAPTER 3

page 70 Top: Makeup Stephanie Neiheisel; model Jess Hause. Bottom: Photography Sara Nevels; model Chante Fox

page 72 Top: Makeup Stephanie Neiheisel; model Jess Hause. Bottom: Photography Sara Nevels; model Sarah Hubbel

page 74 Top: Makeup Aeni Domme; model Lauren Garcia. Bottom: Hair Demi Walsh; makeup Stephanie Neiheisel; model Karra Labombarde

page 76 Top: Hair Walker; makeup Morgan Teresa; model Britnee Penson. Bottom: Hair Genevieve Reber; makeup Stephanie Neiheisel; model Megan Tankeh

page 78 Top: Makeup Stephanie Neiheisel; model Brooke Barker. Bottom: Makeup Stephanie Neiheisel; model Talina Talburt

page 80 Top: Hair Anthony Lunam; makeup Stephanie Neiheisel; model Megan Tankeh. Bottom: Hair Anthony Lunam; makeup Stephanie Neiheisel; model Courtney Larsen

page 82 Top: Hair Tracy Melton; makeup Tracy Melton; photography Danielle M. Sabol. Bottom: Hair Anthony Lunam; makeup Stephanie Neiheisel

page 84 Top: Makeup Stephanie Neiheisel; model Jess Hause. Bottom left: Makeup Morgan Teresa; model Sungwook O Franke. Bottom right; Hair Molly Gee Designs; makeup Molly Gee Designs; photography Adam & Alli photography.

page 86 Top: Makeup Aeni Domme; model Angelica Karamooz. Bottom: Makeup Stephanie Neiheisel; model Jessica Sarceda

page 88 Top: Hair Walker; makeup Morgan Teresa; model Britnee Penson. Bottom: Hair Anthony Lunam; makeup Aeni Domme; model Dorthy Ha

page 90 Top: Hair Hair Dreams; photography Maria Bradshaw; model Hair Dreams. Bottom left: Hair Missy Sue; photography Missy Sue; model Missy Sue. Bottom right: Hair Ulrika Edler; photography Ulrika Edler; model Ulrika Edler

INDEX

ACKNOWLEDGMENTS

Writing this book has been one of the greatest achievements of my professional career, but it wouldn't have become a reality without the help of some incredible people.

First, I'd like to acknowledge my wonderful husband (and number-one fan), Casey, whose constant love and support have been my rock during this entire process. To my beautiful children, Magnolia and Indy, words alone cannot express how much your patience and encouragement have assisted me. I am immensely grateful. I also want to thank my mother-in-law, Sue, for being my go-to grandma and helping out with the kids, as well as my mum Vicky for being all ears when I needed her the most.

To my publisher Isheeta at Rotovision, your direction, vision, understanding, and belief in me from day one have been a huge inspiration. You gave me the motivation to create this book. But none of this would have been possible without the constant encouragement from Cath, my ever so wonderful editor. You pushed me beyond what I even thought I was capable of and I wouldn't be here without your guidance. For that I am indebted to you.

Thank you also to my clients who have stuck by me over the years, always believing in me and encouraging me to go for my dreams. I want to thank my fans who drive me daily to be the best at what I do; I really wouldn't be where I am today without you.

A massive thank-you to my photographer and friend Tiffany Egbert for working like crazy with me during the very, very long days shooting hair. If it wasn't for you and your magic eyes behind the camera, this wouldn't be the beautiful, eye-pleasing book I see before me. Special thanks to the crew from Tremaine Ranch, Cindy and David Williamson as well as Leah and Matt Theodosis, for allowing us to take pictures at your beautiful ranch. I'd also like to thank my gorgeous models, talented makeup artists, and hair assistants. You all rock!